The Ageing Population
Burden or Challenge?

Edited by

Nicholas Wells
Associate Director of the Office of Health Economics

and

Charles Freer
General Practitioner and
Senior Lecturer in Primary Health Care
University of Southampton

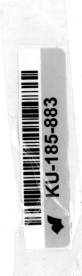

M
STOCKTON
PRESS

First published 1988

Published by
THE MACMILLAN PRESS LTD
Houndmills, Basingstoke, Hampshire RG21 2XS
and London
Companies and representatives
throughout the world

Printed in Great Britain by
Camelot Press Ltd,
Southampton

British Library Cataloguing in Publication Data
The Ageing population: burden or challenge?
1. Aged — Great Britain — Social
conditions
I. Wells, N. E. J.   II. Freer, C. B.
305.2'6'0941   HQ1064.G7
ISBN 0–333–42920–6
ISBN 0–333–45313–1 Pbk

Published in the United States and Canada by Stockton Press
15 East 26th Street, New York, NY 10010

Library of Congress Cataloging-in-Publication Data
The Ageing population.
Includes index.
1. Aged—Medical care—Great Britain. 2. Aged—
Services for—Great Britain. 3. Aged—Great Britain—
Social conditions.   I. Wells, Nicholas E. J.
II. Freer, Charles, 1944–   [DNLM: 1. Aged.
2. Health Services for the Aged—Great Britain.
3. Social Conditions—Great Britain. WT 30 A2645]
RA564.8.A383   1988   362.1'9897'00941   87–18120
ISBN 0–935859–23–3 (Stockton)

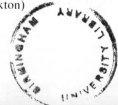

Contents

Contents

The Contributors

Dr M. A. Abrams,
Formerly Head of Research,
  Age Concern England,
12 Pelham Square,
Brighton,
Sussex BN1 4ET

Dr M. R. Alderson,
Formerly Chief Medical
  Statistician,
Office of Population Censuses and
  Surveys,
Medical Statistics Division,
St. Catherines House,
10 Kingsway,
London WC2 6JP

Professor T. H. D. Arie,
Consultant Psychiatrist
  and Professor of Health Care
  of the Elderly,
University of Nottingham,
Queen's Medical Centre,
Clifton Boulevard,
Nottingham NG7 2UK

M. R. Bury,
Sociologist and Lecturer in
  Sociology
Department of Social Policy and
  Social Science,
Medical Sociology Section,
Royal Holloway and Bedford New
  College,
11 Bedford Square,
London WC1B 3RA

Dr D. J. Challis
Social Worker, Senior Research
  Fellow and Assistant Director,
Personal Social Services
  Research Unit,
University of Kent,
Cornwallis Building,
Canterbury,
Kent CT2 7NF

Professor B. P. Davies,
Professor of Social Policy
  and Director,
Personal Social Services
  Research Unit,
University of Kent,
Cornwallis Building,
Canterbury,
Kent CT2 7NF

Dr C. B. Freer
General Practitioner and Senior
  Lecturer in Primary Health
  Care,
Faculty of Medicine,
University of Southampton,
Aldermoor Health Centre,
Aldermoor Close,
Southampton SO1 6ST

Dr. J. A. M. Gray,
Community Physician,
Oxfordshire Health Authority,
The Radcliffe Infirmary,
Oxford OX2 6HE

Professor M. R. P. Hall,
Formerly Honorary Consultant
  Physician in Geriatric Medicine,
Southampton and South-West
  Hampshire Health District, and
Professor of Geriatric Medicine,
University of Southampton,
Southampton General Hospital,
Tremona Road,
Southampton,
Hants SO9 4XY

D. B. Hobman,
Formerly Director Age
  Concern England,
Robinswood,
Georges Lane,
Storrington,
Nr Pulborough,
West Sussex RH20 3JH

Professor B. Jennett,
Professor of Neurosurgery,
Institute of Neurological Sciences,
Glasgow G51 4TF

W. A. Laing,
Economist and Senior Partner,
Laing and Buisson,
Health Care Consultants,
1 Perren Street,
London NW5 3ED

Dr K. A. Luker,
Health Visitor/District Nurse and
Lecturer in Research Methods,
Department of Nursing,
University of Manchester,
Stopford Building,
Oxford Road,
Manchester M13 9PT

Professor A. K. Maynard,
Economist and Director,
Centre for Health Economics,
University of York,
York YO1 5DD

Professor P. H. Millard,
Consultant in Geriatric Medicine
  and Eleanor Peel Professor
  of Geriatric Medicine,
St. George's Hospital
  Medical School,
Cranmer Terrace,
Tooting,
London SW17 0RE

Dr S. M. Peace,
Social Geographer and Research
  Associate,
Centre for Environmental and
  Social Studies in Ageing,
Polytechnic of North London,
Ladbroke House,
Highbury Grove,
London N5 2AD

Professor R. C. Taylor,
Sociologist and Professor of Social
  Administration and Social Work
University of Glasgow,
Lilybank House,
Bute Gardens,
Glasgow G12 8RT

N. E. J. Wells,
Economist and Associate Director,
Office of Health Economics,
12 Whitehall,
London SW1A 2DY

Professor E. I. Williams,
General Practitioner and Professor
  in General Practice,
University of Nottingham,
Queen's Medical Centre,
Clifton Boulevard,
Nottingham NG7 2UH

K. G. Wright,
Economist and Senior
  Research Fellow,
Centre for Health Economics,
University of York,
York YO1 5DD

Acknowledgements

The editors would like to express their gratitude to Desmond Gill for drawing their attention to the quotations with which the book begins and ends. They would also like to thank Maureen Smith and Rita Maddison for their secretarial assistance.

Foreword

Tom Arie

Old age, and even extreme old age, for the first time in the history of the human race, have become commonplace; and this has happened during the lifetimes of those who are now old. Rapid change taxes the adaptive capacity of society, even as it does that of individuals. This book is about these changes, their consequences and society's still imperfect ways of adapting to them.

I knew this would be a good book, and reading it has not disappointed me. When I was asked to write a foreword, I saw that most of the proposed contributors were well known to me, and I remembered Nicholas Wells's admirable booklet on *Dementia in Old Age*, produced for the Office of Health Economics in 1979. That had seemed to me to be a *tour de force*, bringing together in an intelligent and comprehensive way, and in very small compass, most of what was then the key material on that subject; we used it extensively in teaching.

Since then, innumerable new questions have arisen in relation to the aged society (and knowledge about dementia itself has grown by leaps and bounds). The contributors have taken a fresh look at many old questions, and seem to me to have tackled the new ones with good sense. It is generally an ideas book, but it is also numerate — not an attribute of every book on old age.

A foreword is not a eulogy and I don't agree with every point of view here; but I have learnt something new from, or been stimulated by, virtually every chapter. The book has another important virtue: although the chapters are individual, and rarely bland, the text has the homogeneity of a planned and well-edited work. This isn't to be taken for granted these days, when many books are no more than unco-ordinated manuscripts stapled together. This, by contrast, is a real book — informative, often punchy, readable and provocative. I wish it well.

University of Nottingham, 1987   T. H. D. A.

Introduction

Nicholas Wells and Charles Freer

Two men in their eighties meet every day on a bench in New York's Central Park. Carter is the janitor of an apartment block. He has kept the job so long because he is the only person old enough to understand the antediluvian boiler that heats the block. The chairman of Carter's condominium stops by the old men's bench and explains that the heating is being replaced by a computerised system requiring no maintenance, and therefore the janitor's job has come to a natural end. Carter's companion, Nat, explodes:

> You collect old furniture, old pictures, old cars, everything old except old people. Bad souvenirs, they talk too much, even quiet they tell you too much. They look like the future, and you don't want to know. Who are they, these people, these oldies, this strange race? They're not my type, put them some place. You idiots, don't you know? Some day you will join this weird tribe — yes, Mr Chairman — you will get old. I hate to break the news. And if you're frightened now you'll be terrified then. The problem is not that life is short but that it is very long, so you'd better have a policy. Here we are, look at us, we're coming attractions, and as long as you're afraid of us, you'll be afraid of it, you'll want to hide us, or make us hide from you. Don't you understand? The old people, they're the survivors, they know something, they haven't just stayed late to ruin your party. The very old, they're miracles, like the just born. Close to the end is precious, like close to the beginning. What you'd like is for Carter to be nice and cute and quiet and go away, but he won't, I won't let him. Tell him he's slow or stupid, OK, but tell him he's unnecessary and that is a sin. That is a sin against life. That is — abortion at the other end.

Some of the sentiments expressed in this passage from Herb Gardner's play *I'm not Rappaport* reflect the widespread, although certainly not universal, perception of the elderly as a 'problem' group in society. Support for such pessimistic views appears to be readily available from a variety of sources. For example, the elderly — numbering 8.6 million people in the United Kingdom in 1985 and accounting for 15.1 per cent of the population — impose substantial demands on the health and social services. Table

I.1 shows that the prevalence of chronic illness rises rapidly with age, as does the average number of days of restricted activity (through acute sickness) per person per year. Associated with these prevalence patterns, it may be

Table I.1 Prevalence of reported long-standing illness and the average number of restricted-activity days per person per year, by age and sex, Britain, 1984. Source: *General Household Survey 1984* (HMSO, London)

Age	Prevalence of long-standing illness (%)		Restricted-activity days	
	Males	*Females*	*Males*	*Females*
0–4	10	9	19	15
5–15	18	15	15	14
16–44	22	22	14	19
45–64	43	44	26	32
65–74	57	60	34	48
75 and over	64	66	45	60
Total	30	32	20	27

calculated from the findings of both the Third National Survey of Morbidity in General Practice (Royal College of General Practitioners, 1986) and the 1984 *General Household Survey* that about 21 per cent of family practitioner consultations involve the elderly. Furthermore, 36 per cent of consultations for people over 65 years of age require a home visit, compared with 10 per cent for individuals below this age.

In the hospital sector, the *Hospital In-patient Enquiry* for England indicates that people aged 65 years and over account for 32 per cent of discharges and deaths and 61 per cent of in-patient days. Focusing on personal social services, the *General Household Survey* shows that 10 per cent of people over 65 years — 27 per cent among those aged 80 years or more — rely on the home help service. Against this background of service usage, health and personal social services expenditure per head in 1985 has been estimated at £530 for the 65–74 years age group and £1340 for those aged 75 years and over, compared with just £305 per head for the population as a whole (Grundy, 1987).

Concern surrounding the elderly also appears justified from selected indicators of social well-being. The 1984 *General Household Survey* found that 35 per cent of Britain's elderly population live alone and may as a result be especially vulnerable to domestic and other difficulties. (This proportion rises to 47 per cent for those aged 75 years and over, and even further to 56 per cent for females in this age group.) According to the 1981 Census, a further 40 per cent of people who have reached retirement age and beyond live in 'elderly only' households, and amenities in these settings tend to be of a poorer standard than those found in the average household in Britain (Office of Population Censuses and Surveys, 1984).

In addition, the elderly are financially disadvantaged compared with many other sections of the community. For example, the 1984 *Family Expenditure Survey* revealed a normal weekly disposable income of £71.68 for house-holds containing a retired man and woman dependent mainly on State pensions, compared with £182.03 for similarly composed non-retired house-holds. For single-person households the corresponding incomes were £40.25 and £97.09.

Projected patterns of demographic change compound the sombre picture painted above. Forecasts based on mid-1983 data show that the population aged 65 years and over will increase steadily until the first half of the 1990s. The following decade is expected to witness a slight decline in the overall size of the elderly population, but thereafter growth will once again be resumed. More important, however, are the demographic trends occurring at different ages within the elderly population. Given the considerably greater demands placed on the health and related services by the 'old elderly', it is clearly significant that while the numbers aged 65–74 years will fall by 6 per cent between 1985 and 2003, the number of individuals aged 75 years and over will grow by 13 per cent and, more specifically, the number of those aged 80 years or more will increase by 30 per cent. As a result, people in the latter age group will come to account for more than one in four of the over-65 population by the early years of the next century, compared with one in five today.

Yet the pessimism that surrounds the ageing population may to a large extent be inappropriate. At a very basic level, there is a demoralising tendency to view every situation from a negative rather than a positive perspective. Midwinter (1986), for example, has urged that emphasis should be placed on the 1980 *General Household Survey* finding that three out of every four people aged 65 years and over are in good or fairly good health rather than on its obverse that one-quarter are in poor health (Table I.2). Even the finding that as many as 22 per cent of people aged 80 years or more develop dementia (Kay *et al.*, 1970) becomes markedly less daunting when it is instead recognised that this means that four-fifths of this seemingly vulnerable age group do not suffer this fate. And surely the fact that the vast majority of elderly people live in the community — only 3 per cent are usually resident in communal establishments — is to be welcomed, even if it is clear that much more could be done to improve life for many individuals in this setting?

Optimism does not, however, only lie in such 'statistical inversions'. The health of the elderly, like that of other sections of the population, has benefited from the application of new interventions made possible by medical and related research. And mortality rates among the elderly, far from remaining static or even worsening, have shown genuine improve-

Table I.2 Health and mobility among the elderly. Source: *General Household Survey 1980* (HMSO, London)

	65–69	70–74	75–79	80–84	85+	All 65+
Health: % in good or fairly good health	80	77	72	72	67	76
Eyesight: % wearing glasses and not experiencing difficulties plus those not wearing glasses	82	80	70	68	55	76
Hearing: % wearing an aid plus those not using an aid and without difficulty	80	78	73	60	66	76
Mobility: % usually able to go out and walk unaided	95	92	87	74	52	88
Mobility: % usually able to use stairs unaided	97	94	91	84	69	92

ments in recent years (Table I.3). The figures suggest that mortality rate reductions have been greatest among the younger age groups, but if attention is confined to the last decade, a pattern of more equal improvement is observed.

Table I.3 Mortality rates per 1000 population among the elderly, England and Wales, 1946–85. Source: Office of Population Censuses and Surveys

Quinquennium	Males			Females		
	65–74	75–84	85+	65–74	75–84	85+
1946–50	51.6	119.0	241.6	34.4	93.2	208.9
1951–55	54.6	126.7	265.9	33.1	92.4	222.0
1956–60	53.7	122.7	239.2	30.7	86.4	212.5
1961–65	54.0	121.3	253.2	29.8	83.6	206.7
1966–70	55.3	115.9	254.2	28.0	77.5	203.0
1971–75	51.4	116.3	240.9	26.5	75.4	193.5
1976–80	48.8	112.5	237.1	25.3	70.9	192.9
1985	44.3	104.1	223.1	24.1	64.1	178.0
% reduction 1946–85	14	13	8	30	31	15

Optimism can also be generated from a consideration of the circumstances of those who are destined to join the ranks of the elderly in the future. Loneliness in old age, for example, might be expected to diminish because of the greater 'prevalence' of marriage: the 1981 Census found that 11 per cent of all elderly women were single (that is, never-married), compared with only 5 per cent of females in the 40–44 year cohort. Rising divorce rates might, of course, offset some of this gain, although this effect, in turn, may be partially countered if more middle-aged men can be persuaded to respond positively to the known risk factors for coronary heart disease and thereby promote their chances of surviving into old age.

Focusing on home ownership, data from the 1984 *General Household Survey* reveal that 73 per cent of household heads aged 30–44 years and 64 per cent of those in the 45–64 age group are owner-occupiers (either outright owners or mortgagees), compared with 46 per cent among people aged 65 years and over. In other words, considerably greater numbers in future generations of the elderly will have a substantial capital asset at their disposal which has the potential for being employed to promote a comfortable and secure existence. In some ways linked to this observation, it might also be anticipated that forthcoming generations of the elderly — prompted by higher expectations regarding satisfactory lifestyles — and their professional and informal carers and representatives will be increasingly vocal (and successful) in their demands for an appropriate recognition of, and response to, the needs that accompany the process of growing old.

The message to emerge from the foregoing is quite plainly that much of the information — at least at a global level — presented in debates about the impact of the ageing population is susceptible simultaneously to both negative and positive interpretations. The reality, however, as Taylor's chapter and Table I.2 above demonstrate, is that the elderly do not constitute a homogeneous group whose increasing numbers may be seen simply as a good or bad 'thing'. Clearly, there are individuals whose needs are overwhelming, but equally there are many others who enjoy a full and rewarding life.

Matching the heterogeneity of the retired population, there are differences of view among health and other professionals about the most appropriate ways of meeting the elderly's needs. Such pluralism is to be welcomed in that it recognises the infinitely variable nature of the care and other requirements of different elderly individuals. The challenge is, of course, to ensure that the resources available for responding to these needs — £10 billion of public money is spent annually on the care and support of the elderly (Maynard and Smith, 1983) — are targeted towards their most efficient use.

The elderly themselves also face a challenge. Life expectancy at different points in old age has been increasing steadily over time, and the data shown in Table I.4 illustrate the extent of survival after the official age of retirement. Yet the opportunities afforded by this 'new age' are not being exploited to their full potential. In part this may be attributed to material deprivation, but it also reflects negative attitudes to old age. The belief that oldness equals illness or at least signals decline has served to widen the gap

Table I.4 Expectation of life in years from selected ages, United Kingdom, 1961 and 1983. Source: *Social Trends*, 17, p. 115 (HMSO, London)

	Males		Females	
	1961	*1983*	*1961*	*1983*
From age 60 years	15.0	16.5	19.0	21.0
65 years	11.9	13.2	15.1	17.1
70 years	9.3	10.3	11.7	13.5
75 years	7.0	7.8	8.7	10.3
80 years	5.2	5.9	6.3	7.6

between potential and actual achievement (Midwinter, 1986). Consequently, in addition to adequate resource provision and effective usage, attitudinal change — not just among the elderly, but throughout the community as a whole — should be recognised as an important priority. In this respect, a shift of emphasis away from the burden imposed by the ageing of the population towards the more positive aspects of the challenge presented by future sociodemographic trends would be a valuable step forward.

This book considers the existing evidence and prevailing beliefs about the elderly in contemporary society. It then moves on to an examination of the wide-ranging issues that constitute the challenge of the ageing population for professional, voluntary and lay carers as well as for the elderly themselves.

REFERENCES

Grundy, E. (1987). *Br. Med. J.*, **1**, 626

Kay, D. W. K., Bergmann, K., Foster, E. M., McKechnie, A. A. and Roth, M. (1970). *Compreh. Psychiat.*, **11**, 26

Maynard, A. and Smith, J. (1983). *The Elderly*. Nuffield/York, Portfolio No. 1

Midwinter, E. (1986). Old age: illness or opportunity. *Self Health (J. Coll. Hlth)*, No. 13, 15

Office of Population Censuses and Surveys (1984). *Britain's Elderly Population*. Census Guide 1

Royal College of General Practitioners (1986). *Morbidity Statistics from General Practice 1981–82, Third National Survey*. HMSO, London

Section 1
The Ageing Population: Burden?

1

Old Myths: Frequent Misconceptions about the Elderly

Charles Freer

INTRODUCTION

It is perhaps only human to be influenced by the worse case examples, and negative stereotypes of older people will be hard to reverse, but to see all older people as being frail, dependent and diseased is a serious and unjustifiable distortion of the true picture. Sociodemographic trends justify society's concern about the impact of the growing number of older people, but for many the prospect of an ageing population is not simply about numbers, since their fears are greatly influenced by the prevailing images of old age. It is likely that when asked to think of an old person, most of us, whether lay or professional, are likely to picture a frail, bent person, slow to move and think and short of memory. More specific medical stereotypes such as incontinence, dementia and deafness are also likely to spring to mind. As with many commonly held beliefs, there is some basis for this one. The prevalence of disease and dependency problems is higher in the over-65-year-old age group, and the frequency of reported health problems increases with advancing years (Abrams, 1978; Office of Population Censuses and Surveys, 1982; Ford and Taylor, 1985).

Over the past fifteen years, particularly in the United States, there have been strenuous and welcome efforts to create a more informed view of ageing. These efforts have been strengthened by the growing research evidence from social gerontology, which, among other things, has provided a clearer understanding of ageing as distinct from disease. Unfortunately, most of what is written in the professional and lay press on topics related to the elderly makes it difficult to believe that these efforts have had any major impact. The titles, headlines and contents of most articles still reflect an atmosphere of crisis, exploding numbers and impending overwhelming demand whenever the subject of the growing number of older people in contemporary society is discussed. A particular illustration of ageism is in

3

the context of community and primary care of the elderly, where many, providers and patients alike, hold a prevailing negative view about the health status of older people and the likely implications of a growing elderly population on the use of services. In this chapter these views are challenged by examining some of the more positive evidence that exists about the health and social status of this age group.

THE HEALTH STATUS OF OLDER PEOPLE

The secular view that older people are likely to have health problems is supported by almost every health survey since the early and influential studies by Anderson and Cowan (1955) and Williamson *et al.* (1964), all of which consistently report large numbers of undetected illnesses and disabilities in the elderly studied. However, the significance of these results for the *health* status of older people justifies closer scrutiny, since in themselves these findings provide insufficient evidence to equate being old with being unhealthy. Such a view would ignore the difficult distinction between health and ill-health and conveniently dismiss those surveys which have found a high prevalence of unreported problems and symptomatic episodes in younger and apparently healthy age groups (Commission on Chronic Illness, 1957; Hinkle *et al.*, 1960). Not all people without identifiable medical problems can be described as well, but it is equally unreasonable to believe that the existence of a medical problem — for example, a stroke or congestive cardiac failure — automatically means that individuals can no longer be considered healthy. Whatever else is embodied in our concept of health, it seems reasonable to incorporate some element of self-assessment of well-being by the individual concerned together with a measure of the individual's ability to lead a contented and fulfilling life. When these types of ratings are examined, the health profile of the elderly takes on a more optimistic shape.

The majority of older people are well and live reasonably happy lives (Hunt, 1978; Office of Population Censuses and Surveys, 1982; Coleman, 1983), and there is no evidence of a significant decline in happiness or life satisfaction with age (Palmore and Maddox, 1977). Additional evidence is provided by Luker and Perkins's Manchester study (1987), which found that over 90 per cent of the elderly questioned rated their health as being fair to good. The results also showed that almost 80 per cent were able to use the public bus service and that only a minority of the total elderly population required assistance to get around.

There are some important differences between these recent studies and the earlier screening surveys.

First of all, the latter set out to identify problems and, like many screening assessments, to detect asymptomatic deviations from normal. The former, on the other hand, have tended to go beyond the problem to assess the functional implications of the problem. There are, after all, many older people with significant diseases such as arthritis who manage to cope and lead very full lives. Simply measuring the number of health problems — for example, the number of ingrown toenails and corns — is liable to produce not just a high prevalence of unmet chiropody need, but an overestimate of the problem, in terms of practical significance. Surely a more realistic prevalence would be the number of individuals with ingrown toenails, corns and other foot lesions which were limiting their activities of daily living?

Secondly, in recent years studies have tended to include the individual's rating of his or her own health. This is all the more important because of the wide discrepancies known to exist between the actual experiences of older individuals and the expectations and beliefs held by other younger adults about the health and related status of older people (Harris *et al.*, 1975; Age Concern England, 1977). No doubt there are many researchers who would feel uncomfortable about the validity of self-ratings, but a large Canadian study has provided considerable reassurance by demonstrating that the best predictor of mortality was the elderly individual's self-perception of health status (Mossey and Shapiro, 1982). Coleman (1983) also refers to the work of Thomae and his colleagues in West Germany which has produced evidence to show that the 'perceived situation is the effective situation for the individual'. Recent studies of older people who visit their general practitioner infrequently are discussed in detail below, but they also provide encouraging evidence that the elderly can accurately predict their own health needs.

A further feature of the 'unhealthy elderly' stereotype is the view that most old people are in a slow decline as represented in Figure 1.1. This belief is probably enhanced by cross-sectional data which show a greater number of chronic health problems in the very old, but this does not justify the assumption that all older people are on a downhill path as far as fitness and health status are concerned. Many older people do not reflect this pattern. The Duke Older Americans Resources and Services research (Maddox, 1981) found that the functional profiles of the majority of older people remained stable, while older men and women in the Framingham study were much less impaired and disabled than commonly supposed (Jette and Branch, 1981). Also in the USA, analysis of the National Longitudinal Surveys database found that although there was an increasing risk of disabilities with age, a substantial proportion of individuals with disabilities experienced an improvement in functional status over time (Chirikos and Nestel, 1985). A recently introduced system of opportunistic screening for the elderly in Aldermoor Health Centre, Southampton, has included the question: 'Compared with this time last year, how would you rate your health — the same, better or worse?' Early indications are that for the vast majority of older people the answer is 'the same', with a small and roughly

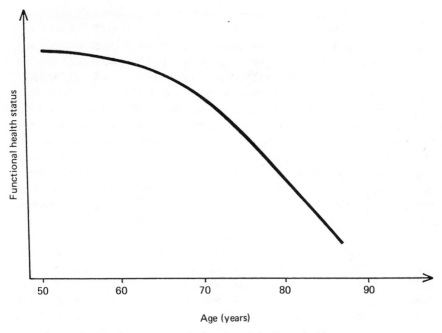

Figure 1.1   Presumed functional decline of old age

equal number reporting either a better or worse state of health. Closer questioning of those reporting an improvement invariably demonstrates that a fresh symptom or episode of ill-health in the previous year had resolved or that they had become 'used to it'. This process of adaptation is central to some theories about what is meant by health. As in other age groups, symptoms are often transient and not every episode of ill-health experienced by older people will herald an incremental decline in overall fitness or health status.

The downward trend shown in Figure 1.1 also reflects the rather simplistic and unwarranted assumption that the elderly are a homogeneous group, a belief challenged by Hunt's survey (1978) and the evidence presented in Chapter 7 of this book. In terms of natural history, it is likely that the elderly are a complex of heterogeneous subgroups, some perhaps showing the slow decline but others the rapid decline of the 'rectangular survival curve' (see Bury's chapter).

The overall pattern of health status and morbidity seen in the elderly will be the sum total of all these individual subgroup patterns of sudden and slow decline, and this may cause the overall pattern for the total elderly population to appear to be one of slow decline. But those who care for individuals of advanced years will know many who have remarkable fitness and good health. These individuals do not show any significant decline with years and may represent an 'élite survivor' group.

LIVING ALONE — A RISK FACTOR FOR THE ELDERLY?

It is very difficult, if not impossible, to find a geriatric textbook which, when discussing the health risks of older patients, does not include living alone. It is equally rare to find any evidence to support this view, and indeed Taylor *et al.* (1983) found that living alone was not a significant risk factor in their Aberdeen study. This probably does not come as any surprise to those who have included a question about living alone in their screening questionnaires for the elderly and found that this contributed to a large number of false-positives. There is, after all, no logical reason why living alone should be considered a risk to health. Over the past twenty or thirty years there have been social changes with the emergence of the nuclear family at the expense of the extended household, and more older people are living alone today — currently about one-third of the over-65 population (Office of Population Censuses and Surveys, 1982). In fact, many older people value their independence, and, far from being a risk factor, living alone may indicate physical and psychological strength. Perhaps our view of living alone is a reflection of societal guilt, and there is no doubt that extreme examples of social isolation always manage to achieve national press coverage. However, most older people living alone have regular contacts with friends, neighbours or relatives (Shanas, 1979; Stuart and Snope, 1981).

When older people begin to find it difficult to maintain their independence, this is likely to be reported fairly quickly to professional services. In contrast, those living with caring and loving relatives are likely to receive increasing levels of support as their functional status declines (Figure 1.2). The relatives may eventually be unable to cope, and the old persons are then in a much more serious and precarious state when they are referred than if they had lived alone. Perhaps living with a caring, loving relative should sometimes be considered a risk factor.

Those elderly living alone are unlikely to be a homogeneous group and no doubt some will be at risk. Feeling alone or lonely is most likely to be a much more important issue than living alone and can, of course, occur when living with relatives. Unfortunately, loneliness, as opposed to living alone, is much more difficult to identify.

FAMILY SUPPORT

A widely heard complaint is that families no longer look after their elderly relatives as they did in previous decades and generations. There have been important social changes, including a greater mobility of the population and a movement away from the extended household. This means more older people living on their own, as discussed above, but there is no evidence that

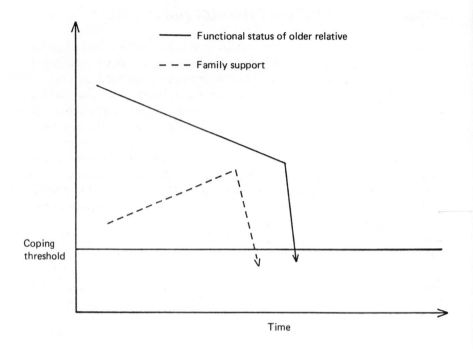

Figure 1.2   The effect of the sudden 'exhaustion' of family support on the functional status of the elderly

this means that older people are shunned by their children and other relatives. Luker and Perkins (1987) have reported, as previous studies have done (Isaacs, 1971; Shanas, 1979; Jones *et al.*, 1983), that families, especially daughters, remain the most important support for the frail elderly. Unfortunately, this might not seem to be the case to those working in health and social services when the elderly present, as they often do, in a crisis situation. At these times, it is usually the case that the relatives are no longer able to cope, but more often than not this is because the relatives have become exhausted after a long period when their close support compensated for the failing health status of the older person (see Figure 1.2). When relatives reach this breaking-point, it may appear to those freshly involved in the situation that the family are not willing to help.

Pressure on hospital and other institutional resources would be rapidly overwhelmed but for the loyal and caring support of most relatives of the elderly with high dependency needs, and while most of them do not seek gratitude, it seems a pity that prevailing beliefs about family care of older relatives fail to recognise the dedication and self-sacrifice of so many caring relatives.

GENERAL PRACTITIONER ATTENDANCE RATES

One of the main reasons for concern about the growing numbers of older people is the likely increase in demand for health and social services; but with regard to general practitioner attendances, what evidence exists to support this concern? It is to be expected, as Knox and his colleagues (1984) have shown, that as the proportion of elderly increases, the proportion of workload related to this age group will increase. But this does not necessarily mean a real increase in workload. Wilson (1982) studied changing demands in his rural practice over 18 years, and could not find any evidence of increased attention required or requested by the elderly.

Table 1.1 shows the general practitioner attendance rates for 1983 in Aldermoor Health Centre, Southampton. At that time the population aged

Table 1.1   Selected consultation data, Aldermoor Health Centre, 1 Jan.–31 Dec. 1983

Age group	No. of patients	No. of consultations[a]	Mean consultation rate	% patients seen at least once
0–64	7578	21 085	2.8	73
65–69	224	674	3.0	73
70–74	252	992	3.9	75
75–79	208	901	4.3	79
80–84	100	472	4.7	86
85–89	45	211	4.7	87
90–94	10	55	5.5	90
95–99	6	49	7.5	67
All ages	8423	24 439	2.9	73

[a] Includes surgery and home visits.

65 years and over amounted to 845 individuals, approximately 10 per cent of the practice population, i.e. somewhat less than the national average. The attendance rates can be seen to rise with age, but the total consultations for this group represented only about 14 per cent of all attendances and visits for the year — hardly a disproportionate demand. It is not possible to generalise from a small, practice-based study, but these results are in line with the findings from the Manchester study of 89 000 consultations (Wilkin and Williams, 1986), which found that the over-75s, who represented 6 per cent of the study population, accounted for only 8 per cent of consultations. In British general practice a high proportion of individuals see their general practitioner at least once a year, and in Table 1.1 it can be seen that in the Aldermoor practice the 65–79-year-old age group reflects the average rather than any above-average pattern. It is also important to remember that higher attendances in older age groups where the total number of patients is small will generate a smaller actual increase in consultations than will similar

increases in younger age bands: for example, in Table 1.1 it can be seen that there are five times as many patients in the 65–69-year-old group than in the 85–89-year-old group.

Ford and Taylor (1985) did not find any significant differences in the consultation patterns for chronic conditions and common ailments between older people and younger age groups. In addition, they could find no significant differences in consultation patterns between the 'old-old' and the 'young-old'. In fact, the 1981 *General Household Survey* showed an overall slight decline in consultation rates by the elderly during the previous ten years (Dowson and Maynard, 1984). If the current emphasis on preventive medicine and health promotion continues, this trend might be expected to continue as healthier lifestyles in earlier years should lead to fitter cohorts of older people in succeeding years (Verbrugge, 1984).

UNREPORTED NEEDS AND HEALTH STATUS OF INFREQUENT ELDERLY ATTENDERS

For some, a fall in consultation rates by the elderly may not be seen as a satisfactory trend. Since the major surveys of older populations thirty years ago, which demonstrated large numbers of health problems which had not been taken to a doctor, the notion of unreported needs in the elderly and the general pattern of under-consulting has been believed to be a problem within this age group (Williamson *et al.*, 1964). In the study referred to above, Ford and Taylor (1985) questioned this view, since their research could find no firm evidence for under-consulting. Of course, there is no reason why the elderly should refer all their symptom episodes and health problems for professional advice. The 'iceberg' phenomenon (Last, 1963) is firmly established in other age groups, and it is to be expected that many of the health upsets experienced by older people will resolve spontaneously, be capable of self-treatment or be of no particular functional significance. Further reassurance is provided by the study from Freedman and his colleagues (1978), who found that the vast majority of problems found at screening either were known to the general practitioner or were of minimal practical relevance to the health and well-being of the patient. This was also one of the main findings of an unpublished fourth-year medical student research project at Southampton (Russell, 1985).

Perhaps the most surprising feature of attendance rates in the elderly has been the consistent finding in a number of studies that non-attending or infrequently attending elderly patients are, in general, fit and well (Ebrahim *et al.*, 1984; Williams, 1984; Williams and Barley, 1985). Concern for non-attenders is the basis for many health screening programmes, and this finding contrasts with the situation in, for example, cervical screening or child health screening, where poor attenders are invariably in the high-risk group.

Russell's student research project (1985) also demonstrated the fitness of non-attenders but, in addition, showed that attendance patterns for high, infrequent and non-attending elderly patients were remarkably stable over five years. If infrequent general practitioner attendance is related to satisfactory health status and persists for long periods such as five years, this may indicate some support for the belief in an élite group of elderly survivors.

MEDICINE-TAKING BY THE ELDERLY

A common medical stereotype of the elderly is that most are being prescribed or are taking too many medicines. Older people do take more prescribed medicines than younger age groups, and some of the published evidence about prescribing in this age group is of concern. Dunnell and Cartwright (1972) found that 92 per cent of patients aged over 75 had taken at least one medicine in the two weeks before their survey, a study in the mid-1970s reported that 80 per cent of elderly patients admitted to hospital were receiving prescribed medication (Williamson and Chopin, 1980) and a number of studies in British general practice have shown that approximately half of all older people take at least one prescribed medicine on a regular basis (Law and Chalmers, 1976; Shaw and Opit, 1976; Tulloch, 1981). Such findings justify the cautions and recommendations in the Report from the Royal College of Physicians on medication for the elderly (1984). However, taking a wider view of medicine-taking in this age group provides a more balanced and optimistic picture. For example, the very high figure of 92 per cent quoted above from the Dunnell and Cartwright study looks somewhat less dramatic when we find that the comparable figure for *all* adults over 21 years was 80 per cent, with the lowest rate as high as 75 per cent; and that in the age group of 21–24 years. Their study could also find no evidence that the buying of non-prescription medicines varied with age. Concern for those elderly patients on repeat prescriptions should not obscure the fact that at least half of the elderly are not receiving any regular prescribed medicines. For those receiving repeat prescriptions, the average number of medicines prescribed appears to be between 2 and 3 (Tulloch, 1981; Gosney and Tallis, 1984; Freer, 1985). My own practice-based study, which analysed drug prescribing over a six-month period in a random sample of 146 elderly patients, found that only 17 per cent of the group were taking three or more medicines on a repeat basis and that painkillers and cardiac or respiratory medicines accounted for over half of all the medicines prescribed. Pharmacologic advances have improved the treatment possibilities for many older patients, and repeat prescribing is not unreasonable in a population where degenerative cardiorespiratory and joint disease is to be expected. Further-more, overenthusiastic opposition to medicine-taking in older people could make doctors and patients feel guilty about their use and thus deny some older people an improved quality of life. There are many patients who could and should be on fewer medicines, but arguments should be based on an informed view and not one that suggests that the dimensions of the prescribing problem are greater than they really are.

INSTITUTIONAL CARE

Probably the two outcomes most feared by older people are institutionalisa-tion and dementia. Anxieties about the former are likely to be aggravated by the recurring public debate about the accommodation needs of those older people unable to continue living in their own homes. In recent years the escalating costs of institutional care, and arguments about public and private provision and how these are funded, have added some urgency to these concerns, which are fuelled by two important but opposing forces. On the one hand, there is anxiety about the adequate provision of long-term residential resources (Grundy and Arie, 1982), and on the other, a general belief that institutional care is 'bad' and to be avoided at all costs. The latter view must seriously sap the morale of staff, relations and patients; worse still, it must add to the insecurity among elderly people in the community, especially those who are frail and fear that 'ending up in a home' is a likely and ominous prospect. Yet in Britain only 5 per cent of the over-65 population are in long-term institutional care, and even for over-75-year-olds, at least 80 per cent still live in the community (Central Statistical Office, 1986). The principle of keeping the elderly at home remains a worth-while goal, but no matter the justification for criticism of the quantity and quality of institutional provision, overzealous concern about institution-alisation must not be allowed to disguise the fact that most older people live and will continue to live at home.

The recent research discussed in Peace's chapter is producing the type of information required to enable those in the public and private sectors to improve the environment offered in institutional settings. More attention needs to be paid to normalising and de-medicalising the institutional environment so that, for the small number of older people no longer able to maintain their independence, institutional care might be a more acceptable alternative than is generally believed to be the case at present.

DEMENTIA

To believe that the prospect of ageing includes a high risk of losing one's mind must be a very disturbing, but all too common, fear. It is wrong for dementia to be considered common in the elderly. The highest published prevalences are about 10 per cent (Royal College of Physicians, 1981), but some studies have found much lower levels, as in the Gothenberg study, where only 3–5 per cent of people of 65 years and over had dementia (Svanborg *et al.*, 1982).

In fact, the commonest mental illness experienced by the elderly is depression, which, though amenable to treatment, is often missed by attributing the symptomatology to dementia (Ham and Smith, 1983). Expectations of dementia by doctors, other health workers, relatives and patients can all unwittingly lead to misdiagnosis and an overestimate of the true prevalence of dementia, as there are a number of important and treatable conditions — for example, hypothyroidism — which can mimic organic brain disease. One fallacy that perpetuates the myth about dementia and can contribute to misdiagnosis is the belief that a failing memory indicates intellectual deterioration. Dementia does include significant memory loss, but the corollary is by no means the case. When busy younger people forget things, it is often attributed to overwork and does not have any of the connotations ascribed to the same level of difficulty in a retired person. For many older people, memory loss for recent events is a problem which worsens with age but without any of the other features of dementia or evidence of organic brain disease.

CONCLUSION

This chapter represents a deliberate attempt to correct popular misconceptions about the health and health care of the elderly. In so doing, it considers the available evidence in a much more positive light than is usually the case. Indeed, much of the discussion about and literature concerning the growing numbers of older people in contemporary society is inappropriately negative, pessimistic and too often couched in crisis terms. Current ageing trends will undoubtedly bring wide-ranging changes in society, but if this is to be seen as a challenge rather than a burden, a balanced and informed view of the likely implications is required. All of the issues discussed in this chapter are relevant to the health and health care of the elderly, and this positive discussion of available data is not an attempt to divert attention from the small but important number of older people who have significant health and related problems. But the lay and professional energy and enthusiasm that will be required to meet the challenge of current ageing trends will not be helped by a distorted view of the situation which exists for *all* older people. Society in general and professional services in particular cannot be complacent, but well-founded concern for those in need of help should not perpetuate common misconceptions about ageing, or interfere with attempts to encourage fitness in and healthier images about the growing population of older people.

REFERENCES

Abrams, M. (1978). *Beyond Three Score and Ten* (a first report on a survey of the elderly). Age Concern England, Mitcham

Age Concern England (1977). *Profiles of the Elderly*, Vol. 1: *Who are they?* Standards of Living and Aspects of Life Satisfaction. Age Concern England, Mitcham

Anderson, W. F. and Cowan, N. R. (1955). Consultative health centre for older people: the Rutherglen experiment. *Lancet*, **2**, 239

Central Statistical Office (1986). *Social Trends, 16.* HMSO, London

Chirikos, T. N. and Nestel, G. (1985). Longitudinal analysis of functional disabilities in older men. *J. Gerontol.*, **40**, 426

Coleman, P. G. (1983). Cognitive functioning and health. In Birren, J. E., Munnichs, J. M. A., Thomae, H. and Marois, M. (Eds.), *Aging: A Challenge to Science and Society*, Vol. 3: *Behavioural Sciences and Conclusions*. Institut de la Vie, Oxford University Press

Commission on Chronic Illness (1957). *Chronic Illness in a Large City*. Harvard University Press, Cambridge, Mass.

Dowson, S. and Maynard, A. (1984). Child consultation patterns in general practice. *Br. Med. J.*, **288**, 1615

Dunnell, K. and Cartwright, A. (1972). *Medicine Takers, Prescribers and Hoarders*. Routledge and Kegan Paul, London

Ebrahim, S., Hedley, R. and Sheldon, M. (1984). Low levels of ill health among elderly non-consulters in general practice. *Br. Med. J.*, **289**, 1273

Ford, G. and Taylor, R. (1985). The elderly as underconsulters: a critical reappraisal. *J. Roy. Coll. Gen. Pract.*, **35**, 244

Freedman, G. R., Charlewood, J. E. and Dodds, P. A. (1978). Screening the aged in general practice. *J. Roy. Coll. Gen. Pract.*, **28**, 421

Freer, C. B. (1985). Study of medicine prescribing for elderly patients. *Br. Med. J.*, **290**, 1113

Gosney, M. and Tallis, R. (1984). Prescription of contra-indicated and interacting drugs in elderly patients admitted to hospital. *Lancet*, **ii**, 564

Grundy, E. and Arie, T. (1982). Falling rate of provision of residential care for the elderly. *Br. Med. J.*, **284**, 799

Ham, R. J. and Smith, M. R. (1983). The confused elderly patient. In Ham, R. J., Holtzman, J. M., Marcy, M. R. and Smith, M. R. (Eds.), *Primary Care Geriatrics*, pp. 137–156. John Wright, Bristol

Harris, L. and associates (1975). *The Myth and Reality of Aging in America*. The National Council on the Aging, Washington D.C.

Hinkle, L. E. Jr., Redmont, R., Plummer, M. and Wolff, H. G. (1960). An examination of the relation between symptoms, disability and serious illness in two homogeneous groups of men and women. *Am. J. Publ. Hlth*, **50**, 1327

Hunt, A. (1978). *The Elderly at Home*. HMSO, London

Issacs, B. (1971). Geriatric patients: do their families care? *Br. Med. J.*, **4**, 282

Jette, A. M. and Branch, L. G. (1981). The Framingham Disability Study: II Physical disability among the ageing. *Am. J. Publ. Hlth*, **71**, 1211

Jones, D., Victor, C. R. and Vetter, N. J. (1983). Carers of the elderly in the community. *J. Roy. Coll. Gen. Pract.*, **33**, 707

Knox, J. D. E., Anderson, R. A. and Jacob, A. (1984). General practitioners' care of the elderly: studies of aspects of workload. *J. Roy. Coll. Gen. Pract.*, **34**, 194

Last, J. M. (1963). The illness iceberg. *Lancet*, **2**, 28

Law, R. and Chalmers, C. (1976). Medicines and elderly people: a general practice survey. *Br. Med. J.*, **1**, 565

Luker, K. and Perkins, E. (1987). The elderly at home: service needs and provisions. *J. Roy. Coll. Gen. Pract.*, **37**, 248

Maddox, G. L. (1981). Measuring the well-being of older adults. In Somers, A. R. and Fabian, D. R. (Eds.), *The Geriatric Imperative: An Introduction to Gerontology and Clinical Geriatrics*, pp. 117–136. Appleton-Century-Crofts, New York

Mossey, J. M. and Shapiro, E. (1982). Self-rated health: A predictor of mortality among the elderly. *Am. J. Publ. Hlth*, **72**, 800

Office of Population Censuses and Surveys (1982). *General Household Survey 1980*. HMSO, London

Palmore, E. and Maddox, G. L. (1977). Sociological aspects of aging. In Busse, E. W. and Pfeiffer, E. (Eds.), *Behaviour and Adaptation in Late Life*, 2nd edn. Little, Brown, Boston

Royal College of Physicians (1981). Organic mental impairment in the elderly: implications for research, education and the provision of services. *J. Roy. Coll. Phys. (London)*, **15**, 142

Royal College of Physicians (1984). Medication for the elderly. *J. Roy. Coll. Phys. (London)*, **18**, 7

Russell, M. (1985). A Study of Low and High Consulters aged 75 years and over in General Practice. Faculty of Medicine, University of Southampton (unpublished).

Shanas, E. (1979). Social myth as hypothesis: the case of the family relations of old people. *Gerontologist*, **19**, 3

Shaw, S. M. and Opit, L. J. (1976). Need for supervision in the elderly receiving long-term prescribed medication. *Br. Med. J.*, **282**, 1672

Stuart, M. R. and Snope, F. C. (1981). Family structure, family dynamics and the elderly. In Somers, A. R. and Fabian, D. R. (Eds.), *The Geriatric Imperative: An Introduction to Gerontology and Clinical Geriatrics*, pp. 137–152. Appleton-Century-Crofts, New York

Svanborg, A., Bergstrom, G. and Mellstrom, D. (1982). *Epidemiological Studies on Social and Medical Conditions of the Elderly* (Euro Reports and Studies 62). World Health Organization Regional Office for Europe, Copenhagen

Taylor, R., Ford, G. and Barber, J. H. (1983). *The Elderly at Risk: A Critical Review of Problems in Screening and Case-finding*. Age Concern England, Mitcham

Tulloch, A. J. (1981). Repeat prescribing for elderly patients. *Br. Med. J.*, **282**, 1672

Verbrugge, L. M. (1984). Longer life but worsening health? Trends in health and mortality of middle-aged and older persons. *Milbank Mem. Fund Q.*, **62**, 475

Wilkin, D. and Williams, E. I. (1986). Patterns of care for the elderly in general practice. *J. Roy. Coll. Gen. Pract.*, **36**, 567

Williams, E. I. (1984). Characteristics of patients over 75 not seen during one year in general practice. *Br. Med. J.*, **288**, 119

Williams, E. S. and Barley, N. H. (1985). Old people not known to the general practitioner: low risk group. *Br. Med. J.*, **291**, 251

Williamson, J. and Chopin, J. M. (1980). Adverse reactions to prescribed drugs in the elderly: a multicentre investigation. *Age and Ageing*, **9**, 73

Williamson, J., Stokoe, I. H., Gray, S., Fisher, M., Smith, A., McGhee, A. and Stephenson, E. (1964). Old people at home: their unreported needs. *Lancet*, **i**, 117

Wilson, J. B. (1982). Workload in a rural practice over the past eighteen years. *Lancet*, **i**, 733

2
Arguments about Ageing: Long Life and its Consequences

Mike Bury

INTRODUCTION

In recent years we have witnessed a veritable explosion of debate about ageing and the elderly in modern society. Sober assessments of population changes by demographers have been accompanied by more emotive statements from clinicians and policy-makers concerning the 'burden' of the elderly, both on the economy and on the social fabric. Indeed, the economic implications of an ageing society have vied with more humanitarian concerns defining 'the problem' of old age (Macintyre, 1977), with fears of a growing 'unproductive' sector of the population raising not a small degree of apprehension among planners and politicians alike. Attempts to clarify the terms of the debate and provide a rational appraisal of old age in modern society, for research endeavours and for policy-making, have been late arriving on the scene. For too long the debate has proceeded as if the facts about ageing population were self-evident, and their implications clear for all to see. These latter have been largely negative, regarding the aged as burdensome to themselves, their families and, not least, the public purse. Even radical analyses, which have sought to challenge a view of the elderly as 'a burden' by arguing that modern capitalism has produced a 'structured dependency' of the elderly (through, for example, enforced retirement and poverty (Walker, 1986)) have tended to reinforce a pessimistic view of the processes at work. Thus, 'relative deprivation', powerlessness and loneliness have been portrayed as the hallmarks of recent experience among the elderly.

From time to time, however, a more positive note has been sounded. It has been suggested that our negative assumptions about ageing can be examined, and even challenged, particularly those regarding health. One such note was struck by Fries in an article published in the *New England Journal of Medicine* in 1980 (Fries, 1980) and subsequently expanded in other publications (Fries and Crapo, 1981; Fries, 1983). Quite against the prevailing mood, Fries stated that his assessment of the situation led him to argue that 'the number of very old persons will not increase, that the average period of diminished physical vigour will decrease, that chronic disease will occupy a smaller proportion of the typical lifespan, and that the need for medical care in later life will decrease' (Fries, 1980, p. 130). This statement, published in an influential medical journal, by an active clinician and researcher in the fields of rheumatology and rehabilitation, was clearly designed to challenge existing suppositions and to throw a spanner, so to speak, into the gerontological and policy works. Although an emphasis on positive aspects of ageing is found elsewhere in the literature, Fries's particular conception of the issues facing us in the future has commanded widespread attention. The terms of Fries's argument have subsequently come under considerable scrutiny, especially by Manton (1982), Schneider and Brody (1983) and Brody (1985).

The purpose of the present chapter is to provide a brief resumé of these arguments, and to examine their usefulness for research and policy-making. After outlining the main terms of Fries's position, and the responses to it, I then go on to hazard some comments of my own, both about the ability of the debate to generate researchable issues and about some of its normative and ideological undercurrents. Against this backdrop I finally make some suggestions concerning future lines of research in the field.

THE 'RECTANGULARISATION OF MORTALITY' AND 'COMPRESSION OF MORBIDITY'

The appearance of the above phrases on the printed page may have already switched some readers off, but I hope not too many. By introducing these terms into his original argument, Fries hoped to draw attention to what he saw as two related processes occurring in modern society (though his own argument is based solely on the USA).

To take the first term first: the 'rectangularisation of mortality' refers to the effect of a fall in the number of 'premature deaths' on the natural lifespan. By 'natural lifespan' Fries means the 'average longevity in a society without disease or illness' — in other words, the average length of life from birth, which might be expected in the absence of illness. By assuming that the 'natural lifespan' is fixed (and Fries argues that it is), improvements to mortality will tend to produce an 'ideal' survival curve, as illustrated in Figure 2.1.

What this means is that, as premature death is reduced, more and more people will live to the limits of the natural lifespan, which Fries claims is fixed at 85 years. At that point the death rate will be so high that it will create a sharp drop in the survival curve, producing, therefore, a near-rectangular picture of mortality. The result of this process, according to

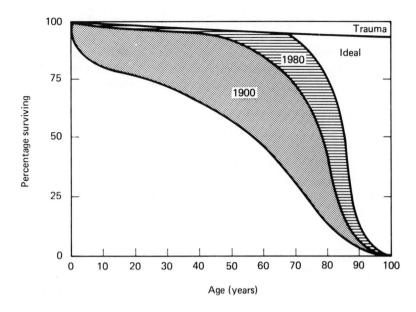

Figure 2.1 The increasingly rectangular survival curve. Source: Fries (1980)

Fries, is the development of 'natural death': the result of the body finally wearing out at the end of the lifespan rather than prematurely being cut down by disease. This point is reinforced by stressing the role of accident and trauma, and the lessening impact of infectious disease, in deaths occurring in early life. However, because some premature death will always occur, if only because of 'biologic distribution' as well as trauma, the 'ideal survival curve will never be completely rectangular'. Nonetheless, for Fries 'the medical and social task of eliminating premature death is largely accomplished' (Fries, 1980, p. 132).

This last point provides Fries with the basis for the second part of his argument. If premature death has largely come under control, especially as the result of the control of infections and the fall in neonatal deaths, we now face a period dominated by chronic disease. Where the river of infectious disease has dried up, 'other waters flow' (Wood *et al.*, 1980). This has implications, not just for the pattern of mortality, but for morbidity as well. For, if the onset of such diseases can also be 'postponed' (by preventive health care, judicious use of health services and increasing personal responsibility), then a 'compression of morbidity' will occur. As Fries (1980, p. 133) puts it: 'The amount of disability can decrease as morbidity is compressed into the shorter span between the increasing age at onset of disability and the fixed occurrence of death. The end of the period of adult vigour will come later than it used to. Postponement of chronic illness thus results in rectangularisation not only of the mortality curve but also of the morbidity curve'.

From these propositions Fries goes on to issue his challenge to current attitudes about ageing. Individual variations in the ageing process, when taken against his picture of mortality and morbidity changes, give grounds for considerable optimism. He states (Fries, 1980, p. 134): 'An inference is that personal choice is important — one can choose not to age rapidly in certain faculties, within broad biologic limits.' Research should therefore examine these individual variations and the causal sequences that create differences in ageing among individuals. With a progressive 'rectangularisation' of mortality and morbidity, a continued emphasis on high-technology medicine 'epitomises the absurd'. Rather than spend time (and money) on respirators and dialysis machines, we should be emphasising human interaction, and argue for a view of ageing which might even be 'exhilarating', given a recognition 'that the goal of a vigorous long life may be an attainable one' (Fries, 1980, p 135). Policy-makers can encourage individuals to take responsibility for their own health and even their longevity (though such responsibilities may be 'painful' for people to accept), and, with a recognition of the changes being portrayed, gloom about ageing can be dissipated.

THE RESPONSE TO FRIES

Not surprisingly, given the deliberately challenging way in which Fries set out his argument, responses soon appeared. Most important were those by Schneider, Brody and Manton, and, for the sake of brevity, it is on their papers that I wish to concentrate (Manton, 1982; Schneider and Brody, 1983; Brody, 1985). First and foremost is the question of the lifespan. I hope it has been made clear that the 'rectangularisation of mortality', in Fries's argument, hinges on the idea of a fixed maximum human lifespan. Claims of longer and longer lifespans were dismissed by Fries as unproven and fanciful, not being backed by scientific evidence on biological survival. Schneider and Brody, on the other hand, argue that biological evidence can be adduced to counter both the 'biologic limit' and 'natural death' arguments. They argue that the ideas that the lifespan of man is fixed and absolute, and that disease is not a major factor in the deaths of the very old (the body having 'worn out' rather than facing pathological processes), is open to debate and cannot be regarded as proven. Manton, in a similar vein, states that there is no clear evidence for the argument that the maximum lifespan is fixed and is now being reached (Manton, 1982, p. 197).

Further, Schneider and Brody argue that Fries's position rests on an assumption that mortality rates among the elderly have reached a plateau. They find this proposition difficult to accept, as mortality rates in the USA 'resumed their decline in the 1970s' and, in particular, a 'rapid decline in mortality rates for the elderly has occurred in the past 10 years'. Even more important, mortality rates for persons over 85 years of age are 'decreasing faster than that of any other old age group' (Schneider and Brody, 1983, p. 854; see also Manton, 1982, p. 192). The fall in mortality rates among the elderly in the USA is shown in Figure 2.2.

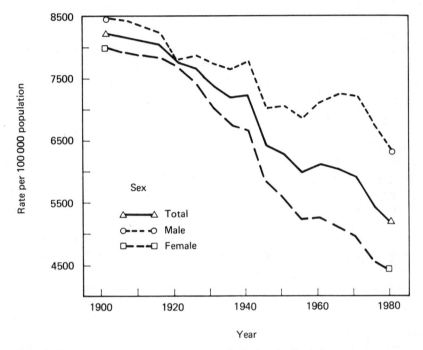

Figure 2.2   Mortality rate for years 1900–79 in the USA (ages 65 and over). Source: Brody (1985)

The growing importance of the 'oldest old' is underlined by these changes. Indeed, Brody (1985) maintains that 'within a very few years about half the population will live more than 80 years'. Thus, the growing numbers of older persons, and especially the 'oldest old', are not simply a function of changing mortality rates at earlier ages. They also represent a change in the mortality rates at extreme ages, which suggests that no maximum lifespan has now been reached, as Fries argues. While these data relate to the American experience, there is a broadly similar picture in the UK, as I shall show below.

Turning to the 'compression of morbidity' argument, Schneider and Brody cast a sceptical eye over the assumptions made by Fries. Here their argument is concerned with whether or not the onset of chronic disease can be postponed. They argue that there is an 'absence of evidence of declining morbidity in any age group, particularly those aged 45–64 years' (Schneider and Brody, 1985, p. 855). Moreover, the 'oldest old' present major problems in relation to health; Schneider and Brody point to the greater need for health services among the very old and the steeply rising proportion of those found in institutional care at 85 years and over*.

In his later paper Brody (1985) points to two further problems with Fries's argument on the compression of morbidity.

First is the term 'morbidity' itself. Brody argues that there is an absence of data suggesting an 'age-specific decline' in such conditions as 'deafness, blindness, hip-fracture, osteoarthritis, and Alzheimer's disease'. More generally, Brody argues that 'we lack methods to measure good or compromised health' (Brody, 1985, p. 464). Routine statistics on recorded illness and disability may provide broad guidelines but they are unable to tell us much about what is happening to changes in health status. Alterations in definitions, in the use of screening instruments and in self-reports may all be disguised by routine statistics, and, in turn, these may disguise changes or continuity in actual experience. Thus, knowing whether morbidity has been postponed or not depends on establishing much clearer definitions and measures.

Second is the issue of prevention. For Fries, one of the key ways in which the delay in the onset of disability or disease can occur is in the adoption of an active and healthy lifestyle by individuals. Fries states: 'I tell my patients to exercise and to "use it or lose it"; "run not rest" is the new advice of the cardiologist' (Fries, 1980, p. 133). As with the opposition to sin, few of us would want to take a stand against health promotion and disease prevention. Brody, however, points to the dangers of overstating the impact of such activities and behaviours on health, and points to the 'crisis of credibility' that can occur when 'scientific evidence is weak or lacking'. As far as the elderly are concerned, Brody argues that there is 'almost no association between most of the commonly advocated personal health practices and mortality among the elderly' (Brody, 1985, p. 465). General prescriptions about diet and exercise, for example, might be attractive for some older persons, but not for others. Few of those living with chronic arthritic pain, the aftermath of a stroke or the consequences of Parkinsonism, for example, are likely to benefit from being told to take vigorous exercise.

Finally, Schneider and Brody (1983) warn against the 'seductive predictions' of Fries as a basis for policy-making. Although they support policy initiatives for prevention, they depart from Fries when he predicts that the need for health care will decrease as morbidity and mortality are 'rectangularised'. In contrast, they argue that 'valuable resources' should not be directed away from the treatment and management of chronic conditions,

---

* The association between age, health service utilisation and need requires careful examination. See, for example, recent discussions by Ford and Taylor (1985) and Wolinsky *et al.* (1986).

and they point to the difficult political decisions that confront a society concerning the quality and quantity of health care to be provided in a situation where 'a huge proportion' will be suffering from chronic disease. In this way the scientific issues inevitably become intertwined with political considerations, with Brody warning that Fries's argument may well be used by policy-makers as a rationale for the reduction in medical care for the elderly. Therefore, in assessing the arguments put forward by Fries, and by Schneider and Brody, it is necessary to consider both the evidence and the uses to which it may be put.

EVIDENCE AND IDEOLOGY IN THE DEBATE

In developing this point let me first return to the foundation stone of Fries's edifice — the fixed lifespan. Part of his argument here is that the numbers of the very old are not increasing — that is, those living beyond the fixed lifespan of 85 years. His picture of an increasingly 'rectangularised' mortality curve involves the argument that death rates are very high at the end of the lifespan, and show no sign of declining. However, even in the presence of high and stable death rates at age 85, an increase in the absolute numbers of the very old can occur (that is, beyond the age of 85 years), as, even in Fries's account, the fixed lifespan is an *average* of 85 years, allowing for a growth in the size of the 'tail' of the distribution, as the proportion of the total population reaching that limit increases. This becomes even more problematic when it is realised that death rates at the age of 85, though high, are not stable or increasing, but rapidly decreasing. Manton argues that as a result of this '*relatively* more of the lifespan is currently being preserved at advanced ages than in the past' (Manton, 1982, p. 196; author's emphasis). In fact, in arguing that the numbers of the very old are not increasing, Fries went so far as to say that 'there has been no detectable change in the number of people living longer than 100 years' (Fries, 1980, p. 130) — a statement which is difficult to reconcile with available evidence.

As far as data on centenarians in England and Wales are concerned, this statement is simply untrue. The number of centenarians has increased ninefold over the last thirty years; in 1951 there were 271 persons over 100 years of age in England and Wales, and by 1981 this figure had risen to 2410 (Thatcher, 1981; Clarke, 1986). The situation of those over 85 years of age has also changed (that is, beyond the point that Fries regards as the limit of the normal lifespan); the numbers have doubled in the twenty years from 1961 to 1981 (that is, from 300 000 to 600 000 persons), with the prediction that the figure will reach 1 million by the end of the century (Central Statistical Office, 1986). Thus, irrespective of arguments about the growth in the proportion of elderly persons and the very old in modern populations (and here arguments about fertility may be more important than those about mortality, as, when fertility falls, the population ages — Alderson, this volume; Smith, 1984), there can be no doubt about the increase in actual numbers, even when one takes into account problems in establishing reliable statistics. From this viewpoint, the main plank of Fries's argument about mortality rectangularisation is found wanting.

In addition to the problems of positing a fixed lifespan and assessing the numbers of the very old, there is also the experience of successive cohorts in relation to general trends in mortality to take into account. Much of Fries's argument rests on a questionable interpretation of recent trends in age-specific mortality rates, especially in younger age groups. Brody noted falling death rates *among* the elderly aged 65 and over in the USA, and this has also been true in the UK since 1970, for every 5 year age group. But death rates by themselves are not a sound enough basis for projecting the pattern of longevity in society. The changing health experience of particular birth *cohorts* may exert an important influence on survival patterns and the total demographic profile. Brody argues correctly that 'we do not have complete data for even a single cohort on which to base projections' (Brody, 1985, p. 464). In fact, he states that 17 per cent of current deaths in the USA are of people born before 1900, and many of the historically specific factors that might influence longevity, both for them and for subsequent cohorts, remain unexamined.

The emphasis by Fries on 'individual biologic distribution' is thus only one factor to take into account in explaining the ageing process. Each generation lives within a unique environment, both physically and socially (in terms of work, lifestyles, stress and social support). Unless such factors are taken into account, predictions about longevity are unnecessarily speculative. Further, it is important to bear in mind that mortality rates may disguise a number of important dimensions of experience. For example, Fox and his colleagues (1985) have recently shown marked social class inequalities in standardised mortality ratios in old age. They show, for example, that men aged 85 years and over with lifetime occupations classified as Social Class V have an SMR of 118 compared with an SMR of 78 for men of the same age in Social Class I. Even if one takes into account the changing size of social class groupings over time (undoubtedly an important issue in assessing patterns of inequality — Illsley, 1986), there are still important issues to deal with here, in explaining the relatively poor survival of some older persons compared with others. These data are also important because, as Brody argues, social inequalities may well influence, and reflect, the availability and use of health-promoting information (Brody, 1985, p. 466). Clearly, prescriptions about prevention need to be seen in the light of variations in health experience within and between age groups, if those who are most in need, or at risk, are to be the centre of health-promotion activities.

Data on inequalities among the elderly, such as these, point to links between social factors and old age which reach beyond the individual level of explanation favoured by Fries. A sociological approach provides an appreciation of the social patterning of survival and the constraints that influence the choices individuals make about their health. From this viewpoint, social position is as important as individual choice. For example, if one considers the impact of gender differences on survival, especially in relation to marital status, the social patterning of longevity may be explored. In particular, there is a tentative suggestion that single women born at the end of the last century may be particularly long-lived (Bury, 1985). This is in line with findings which show that while marriage acts overall as a protector against morbidity and mortality, it does so more for men than for women (Gove, 1973).

Thus, differences in survival between men and women can usefully be explored with reference to *social* as well as individual or biological dimensions of experience. At the very least, the relatively poor survival rates of males in their late middle years warn against an over-generalised picture of mortality 'rectangularisation'. Fries's argument that 'premature death' is now a thing of the past requires qualification. Recent evidence in Britain suggests that life expectancy for men at ages 45 and 50 is improving very little, and for some groups it may not be improving at all (Powles, 1978; Central Statistical Office, 1986; Marmot and McDowall, 1986). It is important, therefore, not to dismiss 'premature death' as a problem, as Fries does, especially when it is recognised that 500 000 potential years of working life are lost each year in Britain from circulatory disease and cancer alone (Office of Health Economics, 1984). Research, therefore, needs to incorporate social dimensions of longevity if a wholly simplified and inaccurate picture of mortality rectangularisation is to be avoided.

Furthermore, the complexity of concepts and definitions of morbidity and disability warns against generalised statements and prescriptions concerning morbidity trends and possible 'compression' processes. Research in this area faces particular difficulties. Manton and Soldo (1985), for example, in arguing for a methodology based on mathematical models of 'life table curves', in order to 'resolve or at least focus the debate on rectangularisation', recognise that any effort to develop this research, especially on morbidity compression, requires the development of a 'common conceptual framework'. As we have seen, however, terms such as 'morbidity' and 'disability' are not used specifically enough at present to allow precise comparisons, contemporaneously, or over time. To be sure, epidemiological, demographic and social research can all play parts in improving our understanding of the factors influencing longevity, but given the fact that the experience and definition of illness are constantly changing (consider, for example, the development of AIDS, or the changes in our perceptions of the symptoms of chronic disease), the kinds of extrapolation made by Fries about the postponement of chronic disease onset are simply not supportable on current evidence.

This becomes clearer if one moves to the level of specific conditions. Both Fries and Schneider and Brody are in agreement that chronic diseases are the most important influence on health today, particularly in relation to the elderly, and this is reiterated in most appraisals of the current situation (e.g. Office of Health Economics, 1977; Wood *et al.*, 1980). Problems arise, however, when one begins to disentangle the various changes through which such conditions might be going. For example, Rowe (1985), in a recent review of a number of important conditions which affect the elderly, documents the changing pattern of need being identified, and definitions being utilised. New diseases are uncovered, or defined in new ways, as with the case of dementia and Alzheimer's disease (Wells, 1979). In the process of increasing our understanding of morbidity in the hope of postponing its onset, there is always a risk (or hope) of uncovering 'new' or neglected areas of need.

The medical treatment of childhood leukaemia, cystic fibrosis and renal failure, for example, has transformed life-threatening conditions into chronic ones; this constitutes an 'extension of morbidity' rather than a process of 'compression'. Not only that: data on mortality for specific conditions show that the availability of health services may not overcome deep-seated inequalities between social groups, including age groups — an issue which is not treated by Fries, in spite of his criticisms of modern medical care. Alderson (this volume) draws attention to the variations in the age-specific death rates for different cancers, as well as quite complex changes in such conditions as chronic respiratory disease, which, though showing an overall decline in mortality, actually show a rise at the younger end of the 60–84 years age range (see also Marmot and McDowall, 1986). Health services may well be able to postpone the onset of some conditions, or aspects of them (an argument which Fries's emphasis on individual lifestyle seems to deny), but it is also true that they must, of necessity, be less effective in some areas, and even at times be implicated in 'creating' others.

There is, then, a dynamic relationship between morbidity, mortality and health services which can lead to an 'extension of morbidity' in some conditions as well as a process of 'compression' in others.

Fries's simplistic criticisms of medical care, and his advocacy of behavioural change as a means of postponing chronic disease onset, do not do justice to the issues involved. Indeed, such are the cross-currents in these respects that general assessments of the impact of health services, and of health promotion, are difficult to make. The impact of coronary by-pass surgery on postponing disability and morbidity in heart disease, for example, is arguably at a different level from the outcome of interventions in lung cancer, which remains depressingly intractable. At the behavioural level, the impact of smoking on lung cancer is easier to assess than the variety of risk factors in the occurrence of heart disease.

Differences of this order cut across the adoption of the terms of the Fries/Brody debate except at the most abstract level. From this viewpoint, the terms 'rectangularisation of mortality' and 'compression of morbidity' turn out to be frustratingly elliptical; intriguing notions to conjure with, but difficult to use in focusing down on current health experience and health service interventions. The health of ageing populations is, in reality, too complex and differentiated to be summarised in this way. While the vision of a healthy and vigorous long life, followed by a speedy and disease-free death, is attractive, it is unlikely on present evidence to become a reality in the foreseeable future. At the very least, the breakdown in organ systems of the body, even if rapid, will surely continue to involve disease and the necessity for some degree of medical management. Fries's folksy image of the 'one hoss shay', which collapses all at once at the end of its useful life, is an amusing metaphor but not a realistic portrayal of human experience.

These considerations lead back to my earlier comments on the impact of this debate at the policy level. In so far as variations around putative biological norms, or within putative biological limits, are seen to be the matter in hand, then research and health education are directed towards the individual. In so far as the individual's membership of social groups remains absent from consideration, it is the 'abstracted individual' that becomes the focus of attention. On the other hand, if the impact of different social environments on health is taken into account, together with the different impact health services may have, then a different form of policy emerges. While Fries's attempt to provide a positive and challenging view of health and old age is to be welcomed, it is important to ensure that his 'seductive predictions' do not become an ideology underpinning the reduction or deflection of 'valuable resources' for the care of the elderly (Schneider and Brody, 1983, p. 855). Exhortations to 'use it or lose it' by Fries may well be appropriate for some elderly persons, but it is important that such messages do not become the basis of a victim-blaming ideology which suggests that health, and even death, are a matter of individual choice (Crawford, 1977).

While it is undoubtedly important to maximise choices, for the poor as well as for the rich and for the old as well as for the young, it is important to appreciate the constraints within which choices are made (Blaxter, 1983). Decisions about health are made within *social* as well as biological limits, and it is part of the remit of health services to act as a buffer against the negative effects of social structures, especially those that produce loneliness and poverty. The role of health services in modern society embodies sentiments of collective responsibility for the well-being of groups such as the elderly, as well as resources for the maintenance of individual health. This is as true for insurance-based 'private' systems of care such as those in the USA (where, in fact, 90 per cent of health service encounters in hospitals are paid for by third parties — Aaron and Schwartz, 1984), as it is in a 'socialised' system such as the British National Health Service. In considering recent arguments about ageing, therefore, the context as well as the content of the debate needs to be taken into account.

LINES OF DEVELOPMENT

As a summary and conclusion to the present discussion, I should like to outline some implications for research which arise from the debate. First and foremost is the difficulty in researching changes in longevity and health status over time. I have already mentioned the attempts by Manton and Soldo (1985) to provide a rigorous basis for modelling the various factors involved, based on a WHO report on epidemiological issues in ageing research, published in 1984. Part of the problem here is, as I have noted, in coming to terms with the nature and definition of disablement. In fact, Manton and Soldo attempt to utilise the concepts of impairment, disability and handicap adopted by WHO in 1980. These try to clarify the basic dimensions of experience involved in the disablement process, and have led to a vigorous debate in the literature (World Health Organization, 1980; *International Rehabilitation Medicine*, 1985; Bury, 1987). However, it is also necessary to take into account the relationship between general health and functional performance, as well as the potential discrepancy between disability and actual disadvantage (handicap) being experienced. What is perceived as a handicap by one age group may not be so regarded by others. Thus, objective measures of functional performance and ability have to be set against the structures of opportunity and the outlook of older persons themselves, and these are likely to change over time. That these factors cut across attempts to construct predictive models of morbidity 'compression' may be regretted, but such processes may certainly become the basis of more focused research. Attempts to compare and contrast measures of disability with self-reports of health have begun to appear and could well be extended (Ferraro, 1980).

In the same vein, the present discussion also suggests that research based on a recognition of 'cohort effects' is necessary when issues of longevity or health status are being examined. The sociocultural as well as the physical environment of different age groups may well affect health, as in the history of smoking behaviour. The intriguing issue which then arises is what basis should be adopted in order to arrive at meaningful groupings. Recently, for example, an emphasis on the 'oldest old' has emerged in the literature (*Milbank Memorial Fund Quarterly*, 1985). In part this has occurred in response to the changes in the mortality and survival profiles among the elderly. For some purposes the 'oldest old' are defined as those persons 75 years and above, and in other contexts the figure is taken as 80 or 85 years. Such divisions are, as yet, largely arbitrary. The demographic 'facts' of modern society simply do not speak for themselves. There is a need, then, for much more debate concerning the health and social experiences of different age groups in order to reach more rational categories, and thus an improved basis for comparative research. In this way the 'social patterning of longevity' might be better understood. Grouping together cohorts born in different environments as 'the elderly' may be administratively convenient but less than satisfactory for the development of more sensitive policies and appropriate research. The presence of considerable heterogeneity among older populations and the need for this to be recognised in research is thus underlined (Walker, 1986).

Finally, this overview points to the need for more 'fine-grained' research on ageing and health. In assessing the usefulness of arguments about 'rectangularisation' and 'compression' processes, it has become clear that the terms used are, in some respects, too abstract to be properly defined or operationalised, and that they rely too heavily on secondary data. When examined, they appear to apply to some aspects of experience but not to others. While attempts to provide health care planners and policy-makers with broad overviews of ageing and health may be helped by these arguments, the present review suggests a more meaningful *locus* as well as *focus* for future research. One of the difficulties with these 'arguments about ageing' is that the data used are too removed from the actual circumstances of elderly people for judgements to be made about such matters as individual health promotion or the need for services. Research needs to be built up from studies of particular communities, their needs, and the sources of support available to them. Of course, representativeness is always an issue for small-scale studies, but without them arguments about ageing will tend to lack substance, and the testing of concepts will remain poor.

Most importantly, studies of health status and the quality of life among the elderly must include an appreciation of the beliefs and attitudes of older persons themselves, and how these vary by generational and other social groupings. Attempts to revive studies of *generation* as opposed to old age alone are being undertaken and could be extended (Williams, 1986). As far as service provision is concerned, we need to know far more about the expectations older persons have of services provided and what their experiences of them are. Against such a backdrop, assessments of effectiveness in objective health status and in such matters as patient satisfaction can be given a firmer foundation. Studies of the very old need to assess how far ill-health and the current provision of services affect not only the individual, but also the closest supporter or carer. Current arguments about ageing cannot, surely, be left at the individual level, as if the elderly are a statistical series, or units of analysis. Older people are members of communities, living within particular constraints, as well as with resources regarding their health and well-being. Unless research is generated on such issues, there is a danger that arguments about ageing will turn from stimulating our thinking to become sterile exchanges between experts on unresolvable issues.

ACKNOWLEDGEMENT

I would like to acknowledge the helpful comments of Margot Jefferys in the preparation of this chapter.

REFERENCES

Aaron, H. J. and Schwartz, W. B. (1984). *The Painful Prescription: Rationing Hospital Care*. Brookings Institution, Washington D.C.

Blaxter, M. (1983). Health services as a defence against the consequences of poverty in industrialised countries. *Soc. Sci. Med.*, **17** (16), 1139

Brody, J. A. (1985). Prospects for an ageing population. *Nature, Lond.*, **315**, 463

Bury, M. R. (1986). Living to be a centenarian. *New Society*, 16 May, 14

Bury, M. R. (1987). The international classification of impairment, disability and handicap: A review of research and prospects, *International Disability Studies*, in press

Central Statistical Office (1986). *Social Trends, 16*. HMSO, London

Clarke, C. (1986). Increased longevity in man. *J. Roy. Coll. Phys. (London)*, **20** (2), 122

Crawford, R. (1977). You are dangerous to your health: the ideology and politics of victim blaming. *Int. J. Hlth Serv.*, **7**, 663

Ferraro, K. O. (1980). Self-ratings of health among the old and the old-old. *J. Hlth Soc. Behav.*, **21**, 377

Ford, G. and Taylor, R. (1985). The elderly as underconsulters: a critical reappraisal. *J. Roy. Coll. Gen. Pract.*, **35**, 244

Fox, A. J., Goldblatt, P. O. and Jones, D. R. (1985). Social class mortality differentials: artefact selection or life circumstances? *J. Epidemiol. Comm. Med.*, **39**, 1

Fries, J. F. (1980). Ageing, natural death and the compression of morbidity. *New Engl. J. Med.*, **303** (3), 130

Fries, J. F. (1983). The compression of morbidity. *Milbank Mem. Fund Q.*

Fries, J. F. and Crapo, L. M. (1981). *Vitality and Ageing: Implications of the Rectangular Curve*. Freeman, San Francisco

Gove, W. (1973). Sex, marital status and mortality. *Am. J. Sociol.*, **79**, 45

Illsley, R. (1986). Occupational class, selection and the production of inequalities in health. *Q. J. Soc. Aff.*, **2** (2), 151

International Rehabilitation Medicine (1985). **7** (2)

Macintyre, S. (1977). Old age as a social problem. In Dingwall, R. *et al.* (Eds.), *Health Care and Health Knowledge*. Croom Helm, London

Manton, K. G. (1982). Changing concepts of mortality and morbidity in the elderly population. *Milbank Mem. Fund Q./Hlth Soc.*, **60**, 183

Manton, K. G. and Soldo, B. J. (1985). Dynamics of health changes in the oldest old: new perspectives and evidence. *Milbank Mem. Fund. Q./Hlth Soc.*, **63** (2), 206

Marmot, K. G. and McDowall, M. E. (1986). Mortality decline and widening social inequalities, *Lancet*, 2 Aug., 274

Milbank Memorial Fund Quarterly (1985). **63** (2)

Office of Health Economics (1977). *Physical Impairment: Social Handicap*, Paper No. 60

Office of Health Economics (1984). *A New NHS Act for 1996?*

Powles, J. (1978). The effect of health services on adult male mortality in relation to the effect of social and economic factors. *Ethics Sci. Med.*, **5**, 1

Rowe, J. W. (1985). Health care of the elderly. *New Engl. J. Med.*, **312** (12), 827

Schneider, E. L. and Brody, J. A. (1983). Ageing, natural death and the compression of morbidity: another view. *New Engl. J. Med.*, **309**, 854

Smith, R. M. (1984). The structured dependency of the elderly: a twentieth century creation? *Soc. Soc. Hist. Med. Bull.*, **34**, 35

Thatcher, A. R. (1981). Centenarians. *Pop. Trends*, **25**, 11

Walker, A. R. (1986). The politics of ageing in Britain. In Phillipson, C., Bernard, M. and Strang, P. (Eds.), *Dependency and Interdependency in Old Age: Theoretical Perspectives and Policy Alternatives*. Croom Helm, Beckenham

Wells, N. E. J. (1979). *Dementia in Old Age*. Office of Health Economics, London

Williams, R. (1986). Images of age and generation. Paper for *British Sociological Association Conference, 1986*

Wolinsky, F. D., Mosely, R. R. and Coe, R. M. (1986). A cohort analysis of the use of health services by elderly Americans. *J. Hlth Soc. Behav.*, **27**, 209

Wood, P. H. N., Bury, M. R. and Badley, E. M. (1980). Other waters flow: an examination of the contemporary approach to care for rheumatic patients. In Hill, A. G. S. (Ed.), *Topical Reviews in Rheumatic Disorders*. John Wright, Bristol

World Health Organization (1980). *International Classification of Impairments, Disabilities and Handicaps: A Manual of Classification Relating to the Consequences of Disease*. WHO, Geneva

World Health Organization (1984). *The Uses of Epidemiology in the Study of the Elderly: Report of a WHO Scientific Group on the Epidemiology of Ageing*. Technical Report Series, 706, WHO, Geneva

3

The Elderly Today. 1: An Economic Audit

Ken Wright

INTRODUCTION

This chapter is concerned with economic aspects of policies for the care of the elderly. One of the major objectives of these policies was set out recently in a Government White Paper (Department of Health and Social Security, 1981, para. 2.1, p. 6) as follows:

> The aim of the Government's policy is to enable elderly people to live independent lives in their own homes wherever possible — which reflects what the majority themselves want. If this is to be achieved, people will need an income sufficient to provide a reasonable standard of living and to enable them to take part in the life of the community. The key to this lies in a basic retirement pension at a satisfactory level, the maturing of earnings-related State and occupational pensions, and any savings or insurance which people may have. In addition, practical help and the provision of care can provide extra support.

There are several economic means to achieve this objective, which are summarised as:

- Providing an income which enables old people to secure a satisfactory standard of living.
- Providing access to a series of services which help to combat loneliness.
- Providing a safe, clean and warm domestic environment.

Each of these ways of maintaining the independence of the elderly is discussed in the order set out above in the next three sections. However, it is recognised that there are limits to staying at home and that for some people, especially those who are heavily physically or mentally infirm, care in

33

residential or nursing homes or in hospital will be the most effective form of care. The fifth section, therefore, is concerned with analysing the costs and benefits of caring for people who are very disabled and concerning whose care there is a continuing argument about the most efficient allocation of resources.

PROVISION OF AN INCOME TO MAINTAIN A SATISFACTORY STANDARD OF LIVING

The source and size of incomes of households whose heads are classified as elderly (60 years or more for women and 65 years or more for men) are set out in Table 3.1. The figures illustrate the usual worries that people have

Table 3.1 Sources of household incomes — retired and non-retired households. Source: *Family Expenditure Survey 1984*, Table 21, p. 61, and Table 23, p. 67 (Department of Employment, 1986)

Household type	Gross normal weekly household income (£)	Wages and salaries (£)	Social security benefits (£)	Other (£)
One man: under 65	136.06	98.91	9.62	27.53
One man: over 65	74.14	1.59	37.38	35.16
One woman: under 60	112.17	81.05	11.70	19.42
One woman: over 60	62.55	2.86	36.76	22.93
One adult, retired: mainly dependent on State pension	40.34	0.02	37.46	2.86
One adult, other retired household	87.36	–	36.89	50.47
One man and one woman, retired: mainly dependent on State pension	71.92	–	64.14	7.72
One man and one woman: other retired household	150.09	16.42	58.47	75.20
All households	197.37[a]	131.00	27.45	38.93

[a] Average weekly income.

about the incomes of elderly people. Single-person households, both male and female, have much lower incomes than their non-retired counterparts. The incomes of the retired householders are around 55 per cent of those of the non-retired householders in both instances. The households, both one- and two-person, which suffer the lowest incomes are those with retired persons dependent mainly on State pensions. These households have less than half the weekly income of other retired households. About 47 per cent of retired households fall into this lowest income category.

As shown in Table 3.2, per capita, the pensioner households do not have the lowest disposable income. Large families and single-parent families do

Table 3.2 Per capita incomes 1984 by household. Source: *Family Expenditure Survey 1984*, Table 22, p. 64 (Department of Employment, 1986)

Household type	Weekly disposable per capita income (£)
Two adults, four or more children	27
One adult, two or more children	29
One man, one woman, retired: mainly dependent on State benefits	36
Man, woman, three children	38
One adult, retired: mainly dependent on State benefits	40
One adult, one child	42
Man, woman: other retired income	67
One adult: other retired income	79
Man, woman, non-retired household	91
One adult, non-retired household	97

worse than pensioner households on per capita calculations. Single pensioners with sources of income other than State benefits tend to be among the highest recipients per capita of disposable income. Given the high element of costs of running a household, such as rent, rates, heating and maintenance, which vary little with the number in the household, it might be difficult to make valid comparisons on per capita bases. Nevertheless, such a basis reinforces the previous point that pensioners dependent on State pensions are relatively worse off compared with other household types in the United Kingdom.

The way in which different retired households spend their money is set out in Table 3.3. Households dependent mainly on State pensions spend 30 per cent of their expenditure on food. The other two main components of expenditure are fuel, light and power, and net housing costs. For single-person pensioner households, 28.5 per cent is expended on these two main items; and for one-man, one-woman pensioner households, 24.7 per cent is expended on the same commodities. For households not dependent in the main on State income, food expenditure makes up 18.6 per cent (single-person) and 20.4 per cent (one-man, one-woman), while net housing costs form 30.6 per cent (single-person) and 20.5 per cent (one-man, one-woman) of total expenditure. Thus, housing subsidies help the lower-income pensioner households to close up some of the gap between their incomes and those of corresponding households which are not so reliant on State benefits. The category on which higher-income pensioner households tend to spend a greater proportion of their income than the lower-income households is the use of transport and vehicles. This picture suggests that the lower-income groups maintain a standard of living in terms of basic commodities of food, heat and shelter (thanks to housing subsidies), but do

Table 3.3 Average weekly expenditure of different household types. Source: *Family Expenditure Survey 1984*, Tables 9 and 10, pp. 26–34 (Department of Employment, 1986)

				Household type		
Commodity or service	One-person, retired: mainly dependent on State pension £	Other retired one-person household £	Non-retired one-person household £	One-man, one-woman retired: mainly dependent on State pension £	Other, one-man, one-woman retired households £	Non-retired household: one-man and one-woman £
Housing: gross	17.28	25.26	21.21	17.35	27.88	31.19
net	4.80	22.84	17.63	9.62	26.44	29.79
Fuel, light and power	6.25	7.34	6.26	8.42	9.93	9.13
Food	11.90	13.89	15.42	21.96	26.30	31.17
Alcoholic drink	0.99	1.62	5.47	2.71	4.63	8.49
Tobacco	1.10	1.12	2.51	3.27	2.96	4.64
Clothing and footwear	1.90	3.70	4.82	4.75	7.23	11.00
Durable household goods	1.94	3.74	6.26	4.77	8.24	13.26
Other goods	3.40	5.06	6.17	5.73	11.94	12.97
Transport and vehicles	1.12	5.47	12.64	4.70	16.07	27.74
Services	5.23	9.89	11.22	6.98	14.94	20.64
Miscellaneous		[0.05]		[0.05]	0.08	0.47
All expenditure groups	38.75	74.73	88.51	72.96	128.77	169.30

less well on items such as travelling and, to a lesser extent, on clothing and services.

This picture is reinforced by the data on possession of consumer durables, as shown in Table 3.4. The most marked difference is in car ownership,

Table 3.4 Possession of durable consumer goods by household types. Source: *Family Expenditure Survey 1984*, Table 3, p. 6 (Department of Employment, 1986)

				Percentage of households with certain durable goods			
Household type	*One car/van*	*More than one car*	*Central heating*	*Washing machine*	*Refrigerator*	*TV*	*Telephone*
One adult retired: mainly dependent on State pension	3.4	–	48.6	47.4	91.3	94.6	52.6
One adult, other retired	24.1	–	59.9	55.7	93.7	96.1	83.1
One adult, non-retired	41.1	2.1	55.9	56.4	90.8	90.2	62.0
One man, one woman, retired: mainly dependent on State pension	22.7	–	44.2	74.5	96.4	98.0	66.1
One man, one woman, other retired	58.3	4.6	69.1	84.7	99.5	98.1	85.6
One man, one woman, non-retired	62.2	18.3	71.8	89.6	99.5	98.3	87.7
All households	44.8	16.5	66.4	81.9	97.2	97.2	78.3

where 3.4 per cent of these households have a car or van. Although television and refrigerator ownership is fairly evenly distributed across different households, pensioners relying on basic State benefits are less likely to have centrally heated homes, washing machines or telephones. The relative lack of telephone and motor car in pensioner households, especially in one-person households, is an important point to bear in mind when considering the social isolation of these people.

The possession of housing accommodation presents a different and rather interesting picture. In this case the elderly are in a more privileged position than the rest of the population. This point is demonstrated in Table 3.5, which shows that 42 per cent of elderly households, compared with 15 per cent of non-elderly households, own their dwellings outright. Although such ownership means that no mortgage payments have to be met, it does not serve to greatly enhance the standard of living of elderly people, because, as

Table 3.5   Tenure of housing accommodation. Source: *General Household Survey 1980*, p. 184
(Office of Population Censuses and Surveys)

Tenure	Elderly households (%)	Non-elderly households (%)
Owner-occupier, owned outright	42	15
Owner-occupied, with mortgage	5	41
Rented from local authority or New Town	41	33
Rented privately	12	11

previously indicated, housing subsidies mean that poorer groups of elderly
people do not pay out a great deal of their income towards housing.
However, if the equity locked up in housing can be released, the income that
is generated can have an appreciable effect on purchasing power and
standards of living.

A study of the needs of elderly owner-occupiers summed up their
situation as follows (Wheeler, 1986, p. 22):

> . . . the extension of owner occupation has constituted the biggest shift in
> inheritable wealth in the course of this century. A source of finance is now
> potentially available for the benefit of substantial numbers of low-income
> elderly owner occupiers at a time when their level of living and quality of their
> housing is deteriorating and the level of public expenditure contracting.
> Although increasing numbers of elderly people will, in future, have access to
> higher incomes through more generous pension provision, growing numbers,
> particularly women, will continue to experience poverty in old age. A growing
> proportion of this latter group will be owner occupiers who are 'house rich, cash
> poor'. New building society legislation and a more relaxed consumer view of
> inheritance provide the basis of unravelling this 'Catch-22' situation through the
> development of home equity conversion.

The development of new schemes to convert home equity wealth into
everyday disposable income, together with the development of better State
or employer-provided pension schemes, holds out a hope for future generations of pensioners to maintain a relatively satisfactory standard of living.
From the data presented in this section, the present generation are
struggling to afford the 'extras' of life — those services and commodities
which add to the basic requirements of shelter, nutrition and warmth.
Poverty among the elderly is still widespread, and basic State pension,
although increasing with the rate of inflation, is not rising quickly enough to
ensure that the incomes of elderly people keep pace with those of the rest of
the population (Walker, 1986). Thus, it is essential that supplementary cash
benefits and services be targeted at ensuring that the most vulnerable section
of the population is helped to lead as full a life as possible in the community,

that their domestic environment is satisfactory and that they receive help to compensate for any disability they suffer. These factors are discussed in the sections which follow.

SOCIAL INTEGRATION

The need to combat social isolation and the loneliness that this produces is a major factor in maintaining the independence of the elderly. The most vulnerable section of the population is that formed by elderly people living alone. According to one recent source, 34 per cent of elderly people live alone (Office of Population Censuses and Surveys, 1982, p. 182) and 48 per cent of people aged 85 years or more live alone.

Despite these figures, the great majority of elderly people have regular contact with friends and relatives. Only 3 per cent of all elderly people had no contact with friends or relatives (5 per cent aged 85 years or more), and 85 per cent saw relatives and friends at least two to three times per week (Office of Population Censuses and Surveys, 1982, Table 10.22, p. 196; Table 10.25, p. 199). However, contact with friends or relatives does not necessarily rid people of the feelings of loneliness. An earlier survey (Hunt, 1978) showed that 33.7 per cent of people interviewed listed loneliness as one of the things particularly disliked. Almost half of this proportion (16.5 per cent) felt lonely on the loss of a partner, and the remaining proportion (17.2 per cent) felt lonely for other reasons (Hunt, 1978, p. 132).

There is no easy way to deal with loneliness and isolation in the elderly population. One way, of course, is to provide suitable day centres and social clubs. Evidence suggests (Carter, 1981) that these centres provide companionship and a quantity of social relationship that the attenders appreciate. However, a quality of relationship, particularly for confidential advice and talk, is the major gap in this sort of provision. Day care is used by only a small proportion (3 per cent) of elderly people at home.

The costs of day centre attendances can vary widely even within one locality — for example, from nil (for use of residential homes where the people attending did not need transport or extra staffing) to £8 per attendance (1977 prices) where people needed specialised transport to, and staff at, the centre (Wright *et al.*, 1981). The provision of day care for severely disabled people is, however, part of a whole range of services, and the costs, as in the alarm system mentioned later, need to be seen in the light of a service strategy aimed at keeping elderly people at home. This topic is taken up later (p. 46).

The elderly themselves seem to favour more home-based facilities. In the survey of elderly people at home, 11.1 per cent of people interviewed suggested visits by voluntary helpers as a way of dealing with loneliness. A further 6.8 per cent suggested visits from voluntary helpers to assist with tasks, and 10.8 per cent favoured regular medical, welfare visits (Hunt, 1978, p. 132).

Loneliness is not the only undesirable consequence of living alone. Many elderly people have great fears about help not being available in an emergency. Many local authorities have developed alarm systems to meet this fear. A recent guide (RICA, 1986) has shown the usefulness of these systems in that:

- They are effective if given to people who are particularly at risk, e.g. alone and disabled.
- They provide reassurance.
- They do not undermine the morale of elderly people or encourage them to be overdependent.

The costs of the service vary according to the type of alarm used. There are no specific cost-effectiveness studies of alarm systems, and this is not altogether surprising, since alarm systems are meant to complement rather than substitute for other care services. However, as indicated previously, the costs of alarm systems as part of a package of domiciliary services are discussed later.

PROVISION OF A SAFE, WARM, CLEAN AND COMFORTABLE DOMESTIC ENVIRONMENT

Safety

The elderly are more prone to domestic accidents than are the rest of the population. One recent study estimated that 6.2 per cent of elderly people over the age of 75 will have a domestic accident in one year. More seriously, 68 per cent of all fatal domestic accidents involve people over the age of 65, and falls in the house account for over 75 per cent of fatal domestic accidents to elderly people (RICA, 1986, p. 4). Although prevention of falls is, on the whole, a medical concern, improvements in the home such as provision of hand-rails, stair-lifts and bathing aids help as preventive measures. The avoidance altogether of the need to climb steps or stairs forms another effective preventive method. Although only 8 per cent of all elderly people living at home cannot manage stairs or steps without help, 16 per cent of people aged 80–84 years and 31 per cent of people aged 85 or over are disabled in this way (Office of Population Censuses and Surveys, 1982, Table 10.13, p. 189). Thus, one way of avoiding domestic accidents would be to ensure that elderly people, especially the very old, were able to manage most of the time without having to climb stairs or steps. This does not necessarily mean moving into specialised dwellings, helpful as this usually is, but ensuring that living-room, kitchen and toilet are on one level, and that, if it is not possible to keep bedrooms at the same level, another toilet is available on the same storey as the bedroom.

Given that the great majority of elderly people can negotiate a level surface without help from other people (even among the people aged 85 and more, 90 per cent can walk on the level — Office of Population Censuses and Surveys, 1982, *loc. cit.*), there is scope to adapt housing to help the elderly to cope with potentially dangerous stairs and steps. The recent study of Anchor Housing Trust's 'Staying Put' scheme (Wheeler, 1985) has shown how some elderly owner-occupiers have satisfactorily adapted their homes using special mortgage facilities. For relatively low expenditures, such a scheme can be spread not only to other owner-occupiers, but also to tenants in either council or privately owned properties.

Warmth

A warm home is not just a comfort; it is a powerful agent in the maintenance of good health and independence. As shown in Table 3.4, elderly households generally are not as well provided with central heating as are other households. Lack of warmth in the living-room was a complaint of 8.5 per cent of the elderly at home, and 50.6 per cent of those people said that the inability to afford to spend more on heating was a contributory factor to this complaint, while 45.2 per cent singled out draughty conditions as another cause (Hunt, 1978, p. 80). The poorest sections of the elderly population are the least likely to have central heating, and they spend a larger proportion of their money on heat, power and light than do other higher-income households, whether they be pensioner or younger households. Although there is provision in the Social Security Regulations to supplement incomes to meet heating costs, especially in periods of excessively cold weather, there seems to be a case for at least investing more money in insulation and draught-proofing methods, not only to make life more comfortable for the elderly, but also to reduce the risk of hypothermia in very cold winters. However, even with these measures, the major cause of lack of warmth for elderly people is the lack of money to buy adequate heating systems and fuel.

General Domestic Comfort

This section is concerned with providing the means to enjoy a comfortable life in one's own home. The major factors involved are:

- The presence of basic amenities — e.g. inside toilet, bathroom, hot-water supply.

- The state of repair of property.
- Help, when necessary, to carry out domestic and self-caring tasks.

These factors are considered in turn.

Presence of Basic Amenities

The elderly are more likely than are younger people to live in properties which lack basic amenities such as inside toilets, bathrooms and a hot-water supply. About one elderly person in nine has an outside toilet only (Hunt, 1978, p. 46) and a further one in ten has a lavatory on the same floor as either the living-room or the bedroom. Compared with younger households, of which 99.5 per cent have a hot-water supply, 91.9 per cent of elderly people enjoy this amenity; and 89.5 per cent of elderly households have a bathroom, compared with 94.9 per cent of younger households.

Thus, the point made previously about adaptations to property is also valid for improvements to property. Again, the investment in the provision of basic amenities would serve to make life more comfortable, prevent illness and disability, and preserve independence.

State of Repair

As with the lack of basic amenities, the elderly tend to live in more disadvantaged circumstances than do younger people when it comes to the state of repair of property. Table 3.6 relates to housing conditions and

Table 3.6 State of the elderly's housing. Source: Department of the Environment (1982)

State of repair	Satisfactory (%)	Unsatisfactory (%)	Poor (%)
All retirement groups	66	26	8
75 years or over	59	29	12

makes this point very well. Since the definition of 'poor' state of repair implies that the property requires at least £7000 worth of work to bring it up to a satisfactory standard, it is clear that a major effort is needed, not only to rectify current defects, but also to maintain property so that it does not decline into an alarming state of disrepair.

Help with Domestic and Self-care Tasks

Compared with the problems about housing conditions, there is a much happier story to tell where help around the home is concerned. The main conclusion to be drawn from recent work is that the elderly receive domestic help such as the provision of meals, laundry and cleaning about the house (Office of Population Censuses and Surveys, 1982, p. 207). The main gaps in the provision arise for tasks such as cleaning windows and other work which requires climbing. The tasks which are not done are those which are considered to be outside the scope of maintaining the internal cleanliness of the domicile. As far as personal choice is concerned, many disabled elderly people would like help with tasks such as gardening, cleaning outside windows and paintwork, and property repairs (Hunt, 1978). These tasks are those for which higher-income households can buy private help. Again, it is the lower-income pensioner households who cannot buy those extras which might be considered by some people as luxuries but which go to make life more comfortable and enjoyable.

In the main, these tasks are carried out by spouses and other relatives or friends of disabled elderly people. The Home Help Service, however, plays an important role for those people who live alone and have no relatives living nearby (Office of Population Censuses and Surveys, 1982, p. 204). The division of labour between social public service and family carers becomes more important for self-care tasks such as bathing, dressing, feeding and help with toileting. Several surveys have shown how this partnership tends to work with the more disabled elderly (e.g. see Green *et al.*, 1979).

Taken in terms of proportions of the population affected by the inability to carry out self-care routines, it appears that there is not a great deal of help required in the community. Only about 1 per cent of the elderly living at home are severely disabled. However, this is a case of false first impressions. Increasing physical and mental disability is the major reason for elderly people having to enter residential, nursing home or continuing hospital care. It is around this seemingly small proportion of people at home and the five or so per cent of the elderly people who are in full-time institution-based care that the major resource allocation arguments revolve. This is the topic to be reviewed in the next section.

THE CARE OF THE HEAVILY DISABLED ELDERLY

As stated in the previous section, the major debates about the resources needed to care for the elderly have centred on the care of the highly disabled members of the population. The key to this debate is the identification of methods of care which provide the most beneficial care for a given set of resources. Thus, this topic is addressed by looking at the relative costs and benefits of caring for heavily disabled elderly people at home, or in residential, nursing home or continuing hospital care. Given that previous sections have been concerned with the provision of a satisfactory way of life for people living at home, the benefits of the other modes of care relative to care at home are discussed in the next subsection, followed by a discussion of the relative costs of care.

The Relative Benefits of Institution-based Care

Institutional care covers full-time care outside one's own home, and encompasses residential (private and public), nursing home (private) and hospital care. The term 'institutional' is used as a shorthand method of covering all these types of care, and is used for convenience and not in any disparaging sense. The performance of institutional care is discussed in the same terms as that of home-based care, which was discussed on the lines of how well it provides a safe, warm, comfortable, domestic-type environment, combats social isolation and loneliness, and compensates for disability.

Potentially, institutional care should be able to provide a safe, warm and comfortable environment, although the definition of 'comfortable' needs further discussion, which is deferred for later consideration. Provided that environmental standards of provision of toilet, bathroom and day-room accommodation are met, together with good standards of cleanliness and hygiene, then those benefits should be achieved. Of course, monitoring these standards on a daily basis is very difficult, and severe problems are usually brought to light by complaints or scandals which only surface on the odd occasion. By and large, institutional care is likely to achieve these environmental standards, but, as shown later, at some cost to personal choice and privacy.

However, coping with physical and psychological disabilities varies within the different forms of care. Continuing care in hospital will usually compensate for the most severe disabilities. The ability of the other forms of care is not at all clear. All forms of care can cope with a certain proportion of severely disabled people, as various surveys have indicated (for a discussion, see Booth, 1985). The major points at issue are exactly what proportion of severely disabled people can be maintained in residential or nursing home care and whether or not people with certain disabilities will be refused admission to these forms of care. The two issues are connected, because it may be possible sometimes to admit a severely disabled person into residential care if the proportion of disabled people usually resident there is small enough for the existing staff to cope. On the whole, one would expect people who enter residential care to be able to carry out most self-care routines, such as dressing, washing hands and face, feeding and toileting. People who need help with more than one of these tasks are more likely to enter nursing homes or hospital or to be cared for at home by a relative. Admission to a nursing home, however, may depend on financial circumstances as well as disability, since there are no public nursing homes (apart from three experimental ones) and Social Security board and lodging allowance is needed to meet the fees for people who cannot afford them from their own income. Even nursing homes will not be able to accept some people who are heavily dependent on nursing care (Wright, 1985).

It can be said that there is a continuum or spectrum of care facilities available which can cope with increasing disability. This does not mean that a person has to move through that continuum as disability increases. Although there are transfers from residential and nursing homes to continuing care wards in hospitals, the major move is often from own home to one of these facilities. There is also a continuum of care in the sense that residential homes and hospitals can offer day care of one type or another as well as short-stay accommodation, for either treatment or respite care. In this way the hospital and residential homes become more integrated with the community and provide a mechanism to overcome the problem of social integration in their local communities.

Some elderly people perceive institutional, especially residential, care as being more beneficial than staying in their own homes, not so much because of its ability to provide care and shelter as because it is a means of avoiding social isolation and loneliness. Some gregarious souls positively seek the company which communal living can bring, even if this entails a sacrifice at times of privacy and the choice over the organisation of daily events such as mealtimes, menus and social outings. Of course, how much loss of personal choice and privacy occurs in different forms of care depends upon the way in which facilities are built and administered. It is more expensive to build facilities which give people their own living and sleeping accommodation. However, given that such capital has a very long life, the actual extra cost per resident when discounted over, say, 60 years of life of the building may well be quite small in proportion to the rest of the costs of care. For example, if it cost £5000 to provide better facilities per resident in constructing a home, the annual equivalent cost discounted at 5 per cent is £221, or £4.25 per week. This is about 4 per cent of the average current cost of a local authority residential home.

In addition, the style of care is important. Different styles of management have been categorised between person- or task-centred and open or closed regimes (Wade *et al.*, 1983). This, in turn, yields different models of care — Supportive, Protective, Controlled and Restrained Models. The Supportive Model is characterised by consultation and involvement of the elderly in the care regime, and on decisions about activities and outings. Thus, it is possible that some of the more negative aspects of care, such as loss of choice or the opportunity of choice, can be avoided by people in charge being sympathetic to allowing their residents choice about daily routines, visiting times, activities and outings.

The other aspect of compensating for disabilities in institutional care is the relief this affords to principal helpers, who can become extremely fatigued and stressed by the provision of day-to-day care of a severely disabled person. There is a growing amount of evidence on the burdens that familial or informal carers carry (for a summary, see Parker, 1985). It has long been recognised that there is a difficult decision to be made at times between the welfare of the disabled person and that of the carers (Expenditure Committee, 1972). The old person may well wish to continue to live at home, although institutional care may well offer better care and a more suitable environment, while principal helpers may feel that they can no longer bear the burden of care. Reaching an agreed decision may well take a considerable amount of professional expertise, advice and counselling, and a thorough investigation of all possible forms of domiciliary and day care as well as alternative forms of institutional care. The relative costs of those different modes may also have to be taken into consideration, but there is often quite a useful amount of difference between the costs of care, as indicated below, to allow an imaginative use of services which may satisfy all parties.

Summarising over the benefits of different forms of care before turning to the relative costs of care, the question to be answered is whether domiciliary-based care can compete with the other forms of care in terms of providing a satisfactory domestic environment, combating loneliness and isolation, and compensating for disabilities at a cost which approximates to the costs of institution-based care.

COMPARING COSTS OF ALTERNATIVE FORMS OF CARE

Starting with the costs of institution-based care, the main category of costs to be taken into account is that of costs of day-to-day management, boarding and care. These costs vary according to the care setting and between facilities of each type. Thus, residential care facilities tend to be less costly than nursing homes, which, in turn, are less costly than continuing care hospital facilities. However, in both the residential and the nursing home sectors there are wide variations in daily nursing costs, even in one area (Wright, 1985). Long-stay geriatric hospital costs are particularly difficult to isolate, because many hospitals have a mix of assessment, rehabilitation, continuing care and day-care facilities which are not separately costed. Taking average costs of hospitals which include both acute and long-stay facilities grossly exaggerates the cost of continuing care.

The second important category of institutional costs is the capital cost of buildings, land, furnishings and fittings. These costs are usually valued at current market or replacement cost, and the agreed sum is then discounted into an annual equivalent value, using the current public sector discounting rate (5 per cent for health and personal social services in 1986). Finally, for completeness, the money that residents spend on personal items of food, drink, clothes, tobacco and other comforts has to be included when comparing these costs with costs of domiciliary care. For many residents, the £7.60 so-called 'pocket money' allowance is the amount that is available for such personal consumption.

The corresponding elements of domiciliary care are the costs of housing accommodation, personal consumption, social and health services received, and informal care. The personal consumption element covers the expenditures set out in the previous paragraph together with spending on other consumption goods and services as detailed in Table 3.3 (with the exception of housing expenditures). Housing costs are included when people moving into another form of care free accommodation which can be occupied by other members of the community. This will be most obvious when people who live alone move into institutional care and free a whole house for occupation by other people. When someone moves out of a shared domicile, the freed accommodation will probably be of little use, and therefore value, to the community as a whole.

The costs of services received from health and social services or other public agencies will vary according to the amount and type of help received. With due care, patience and hard work, it is possible to develop unit costs for all the health and social services, so that the total cost of care per period can be calculated for any individual, provided that information is available on the services received (Wright *et al.*, 1981). Costing informal care services, on the other hand, is a much less developed and more haphazard affair. Several approaches have been tried, without one achieving universal acceptance or usage. There are several suggestions to be made about possible methods of valuing informal care, such as the use of the costs of similar public services, lost earnings or lost leisure time, as used in the valuation of travelling time (Leitch, 1978), and the value of invalid care allowance. The problem is that the heterogeneity of the circumstances in which principal helpers carry out their tasks defies the use of one value.

This is not the place to enter into a long methodological discussion about measuring costs. Instead a short-cut is proposed which highlights not just the problem of measuring the costs of formal and informal care, but also the problem of sharing the burden of care between the State and the family.

The relative costs of different forms of care (at 1984 prices) are taken as a starting point. We have seen from Table 3.3 that the weekly expenditure on non-housing goods and services per pensioner household dependent on State pension is as follows:

One-person	One-man and one-woman
£33.95	£63.34

Table 3.3 also showed that weekly gross housing costs are £17.28 for one-person households. Thus, without any services, the basic cost of care (housing — for people who live alone — plus general expenditure) is around £51 per week for one-person households and £63 per week for one-man and one-woman households. The weekly costs of local authority residential care (England and Wales average) were as follows:

	£/week
Capital cost[a]	20
Running cost[b]	107
Personal consumption	7
Total	134

[a] Based on replacement cost.
[b] Based on CIPFA 1984/85 data (CIPFA, 1986).

The weekly cost of long-stay hospital care varies enormously and it is difficult to obtain a national average. Therefore, the figures are used for a typical long-stay hospital taken from a local study of alternative costs of care (Wright, 1985).

	£/week
Capital cost[a]	22
Running cost	190
Personal consumption	7
Total	219

[a] Based on cost of improving an existing building.

From these figures it can be seen that the cost difference between residential care and the basic costs of living at home for someone living alone is £83 per week. If that person is insecure, lonely or as physically disabled as most people who are admitted to residential care, then the question to be answered is whether it is possible to provide a set of services which cost £83 per week or less and relieve his or her anxieties to such an extent that staying at home is the preferred option. If this is possible, then it will be cost-effective to prescribe and deliver that set of services. Similarly, the difference between hospital costs and costs of living at home with a spouse are £156 per week. If that person can be maintained to his or her and the principal helpers' satisfaction for a set of services costing £156 per week or less, then again domiciliary care is the efficient choice.

There is now evidence that imaginatively provided innovatory community care schemes, supplemented by a package of traditional domiciliary and day-care services, can satisfactorily maintain elderly people in their own homes within the cost constraints set out above (Tinker, 1984). These new schemes include features such as specialised housing, radio alarm systems, and the provision of personal help from visiting wardens, neighbourly helps and good neighbours. The weekly cost of a typical set of services (at 1981/82 prices), including all supporting services, varied from £127 to £76 per week (Tinker, 1984, p. 120).

There are other examples of community care service (Challis and Davies, 1980) and augmented nursing services (Gibbins *et al.*, 1982) which also show that cost-effective care can be delivered to maintain people in their own homes. This is not to deny that there will be instances where care at home is no longer desirable. The point of identifying the cost differences between community and institutional care is that they indicate that there ought to be a thorough investigation of the use of intensive domiciliary care packages before anyone is admitted to full-time care. All areas of the country may not yet be equipped to deliver such packages, but the growing amount of evidence of the success of these schemes suggests that it will not be long before they become more widespread.

This is true, too, for elderly people entering private residential or nursing home care. While it is possible to welcome the development of private care in the sense that it provides greater opportunity for choice, even for lower-income elderly people who are assisted by social security, it would be a pity if these facilities and the consequent public expenditure took money or real resources away from effective community care schemes.

All in all, then, there is a wide variety of alternative forms of care for very disabled elderly people and their principal helpers. Thus, no health or local authority now has any excuse for not developing a range of appropriate services, either community- or institution-based, which covers a whole spectrum of demands and provides advice and counselling which guides people to use those services which are most suited to their needs.

CONCLUSION

Since 'the elderly' form a heterogeneous set of people spanning 30 or more years, it is as difficult to generalise about their economic state as any other age group in the population over a similar age range. This brief review of the economic condition of the elderly has nevertheless found several points of encouragement, including:

- A general ability to afford the necessities of life.
- High rates of house ownership, which provides not only good accommodation, but also the opportunity to turn accumulated wealth into supplementary income.
- Compensation for disability in tasks of daily living.
- Development of new schemes to care for very disabled people.

Balanced against these points it has to be remembered that:

- A large proportion of elderly people are among the poorest section of the whole population.
- The elderly are more likely than other age groups to live in dwellings which are draughty, cold, lacking in basic amenities and in a poor state of repair.
- A large proportion of elderly people suffer from loneliness.
- The development of new community care schemes is unevenly distributed throughout the country; many elderly people are still likely to enter institutional care because of a shortage of appropriate domiciliary care.

It is to be hoped that future policy initiatives will be aimed at increasing the incomes of elderly people relative to the rest of the population so that those dependent on State benefits may be able to afford a better standard of living and that health and local authorities will be encouraged to work together to provide good standards of care, either at home or in institutions, for the very disabled elderly people and their principal helpers.

ACKNOWLEDGEMENTS

The author acknowledges the research grant from the Department of Health and Social Security which funds the post of Senior Research Fellow in the Centre for Health Economics at the University of York. He also acknowledges the permission to reproduce Tables 3.1, 3.2, 3.3, 3.4 and 3.5 received from the Controller of Her Majesty's Stationery Office.

All interpretations of the data and any errors are the sole responsibility of the author.

REFERENCES

Booth, T. (1985). *Home Truths — Old People's Homes and the Outcome of Care.* Gower Press, Aldershot
Carter, J. (1981). *Day Services for Adults.* Allen and Unwin, London

Challis, D. and Davies, B. (1980). A new approach to community care for the elderly. *Br. J. Soc. Wk*, **10**, 1

CIPFA (Chartered Institute of Public Finance and Accountancy) (1986). *Personal Social Services Statistics 1984–85*. CIPFA, London

Department of Employment (1986). *Family Expenditure Survey 1984*. HMSO, London

Department of the Environment (1982). *English House Condition Survey 1981*. HMSO, London

Department of Health and Social Security (1981). *Growing Older*. HMSO, London

Expenditure Committee (1972). Eighth Report: *Relationship of Expenditure to Needs*, Session 1971–72. HMSO, London

Gibbins, F., Lee, M., Davison, P. R., O'Sullivan, P., Hutchinson, M. and Murphy, D. R. (1982). Augmented home nursing as an alternative to hospital care for chronic elderly invalids. *Br. Med. J.*, **284**, 330

Green, S., Creese, A. and Kaufert, J. (1979). Social support and government policy on services for the elderly. *Soc. Pol. Admin.*, **13**, 210

Hunt, A. (1978). *The Elderly at Home*. HMSO, London

Leitch, Sir G. (1978). *Report of the Advisory Committee on Trunk Road Assessment*. HMSO, London

Office of Population Censuses and Surveys (1982). *General Household Survey 1980*. HMSO, London

Parker, G. (1985). *With Due Care and Attention*. Family Studies Centre, London

RICA (Research Institute for Consumer Affairs) (1986). *Dispersed Alarms — A Guide for Organisations Installing Systems RKA*. RICA, London

Tinker, A. (1984). *Staying at Home: Helping Elderly People*. HMSO, London

Wade, B., Sawyer, L. and Bell, J. (1983). *Dependency with Dignity*, Occasional Papers on Social Administration No. 68. Bedford Press, London

Walker, A. (1986). In Phillipson, C. and Walker, A. (Eds.), *Ageing and Social Policy*, pp. 184–216. Gower Press, Aldershot

Wheeler, R. (1985). *Don't Move: We've Got You Covered*. Institute of Housing, London

Wheeler, R. (1986). *The Needs of Elderly Owner Occupiers*. Building Societies Association, London

Wright, K. (1985). Long-term care for the elderly: public versus private. *Publ. Money*, **5** (1)

Wright, K., Cairns, J. A. and Snell, M. C. (1981). *Costing Care*. University of Sheffield Monographs, Sheffield

4

The Elderly Today. 2: A Social Audit

Mark Abrams

INTRODUCTION

I shall use the description 'social' primarily to refer to behaviour by the elderly person which involves him or her, directly or indirectly, with other people. The importance of such interaction to elderly people was spelt out by Freud just over sixty years ago (in 1926), when in Vienna he addressed a group of non-medical people who had come together to celebrate his seventieth birthday. He recalled a theme he first enunciated in his middle 60s, which he spelt out more explicitly in 1930 in his book *Civilisation and its Discontents* (Freud, 1973). He then wrote:

> We are threatened with suffering from three directions: from our own body, which is doomed to decay and dissolution and which cannot even do without pain and anxiety as warning signals; from the external world which may rage against us with overwhelming and merciless forces of destruction; and finally from our relations with other human beings. The suffering which comes from this last source is perhaps more painful to us than any other . . . . Against the suffering which may come upon one from human relationships the readiest safeguard is voluntary isolation, keeping oneself aloof from other people . . . . There is, indeed, another and better path to happiness — that of becoming a member of the human community.

The message came across just as clearly a few years ago when, in a survey carried out by the present writer, a sample of 1660 people aged 65 or more were asked: 'What would you say makes life really pleasant and satisfying for people of your age?' Both men and women, both younger elderly (aged 65–74) and older elderly (aged 75 or more), put at the top of the necessary conditions 'having good friends and good neighbours'. This came well ahead of 'good health' and 'enough money', and its lead, while common both to those who lived alone and those who lived with others, was a little more marked among the former. In a follow-up question, respondents were asked, irrespective of what condition they had given as most important,

'Would you say that you have this to a great extent, to a certain extent, hardly at all, or not at all?' Of those who had nominated 'good friends and neighbours', one-half (51 per cent) said that they had this to a great extent and one-third (34 per cent) said that they had this to a certain extent (Abrams, 1978).

The prescription of good friends and neighbours as a condition for a satisfying old age was, in a sense, validated when the original respondents were reinterviewed after a lapse of three years. As a first step, all the original respondents were allotted a position (low, medium, high) on a social interaction scale. The extent of each person's social interaction in 1977 was calculated by allotting him* one point for a positive answer regarding each of the following four events:

- Received visits at least once a week from friends and kin.
- Visited friends and kin at least once a week.
- Said they had all the good friends anyone could wish.
- Said they had someone to talk to about personal things.

Among those with minimal social interaction (that is, with scores of 0 or 1), the death rate over the three years was 41 per cent; among the rest of the male sample, the death rate was 22 per cent.

A second scale used in the survey sought to distinguish between those who were isolated and those who were not. This scale had eight items. An 'isolation point' was allotted for the endorsement in 1977 of each of the following:

- Had no close friends living in or near the respondent's district.
- Never went to church/chapel/synagogue for any purpose — religious or social.
- Had no living brothers or sisters.
- Had never had any children.
- Was never visited by friends or relatives.
- Never paid visits to friends or relatives.
- Had had no visitors of any kind during the weekend preceding the interview.
- Belonged to no clubs or societies.

Of all male respondents, 22 per cent had high isolation scores — that is, said that at least five of these conditions applied to themselves. Three years later, 30 per cent of these 'isolates' were dead; among those with low isolation

---

* Almost all of those who had died between 1977 and 1980 were men; the figures at this stage are therefore restricted to the men interviewed in 1977.

scores the death rate was little more than half this figure — only 17 per cent (Abrams, 1981).

HOLIDAYS AND SPORTS ACTIVITIES

In recent years contacts with 'secondary' groups have tended to increase. For example, the holiday market has shown an increasing interest in providing holidays for the elderly, and, partly as a result of the energetic marketing of holidays to this section of the population, the proportion of elderly people who take at least one holiday each year has grown substantially.

Throughout 1985, The National Readership Survey interviewed a sample of 5300 people aged 65 years or more and asked them whether they had taken any holidays (a holiday was defined as a break of four or more nights away from home) during the last twelve months before being interviewed. Half of them said that they had, and almost half of these holiday-takers had taken two or more holidays during the year. Three-quarters of all holidays had been taken somewhere in Britain, but almost 20 per cent had involved travel to the Continent — mainly to Mediterranean resorts. In Table 4.1 the holidays of the elderly are compared with those of the middle-aged — the most prosperous section of the population. The gap between the two age bands is not as great as one might have thought, given the difference between the two in income, physical health and mobility.

Table 4.1 Holidays taken in past 12 months

	Men		Women	
	45–64 (%)	*65 or over (%)*	*45–64 (%)*	*65 or over (%)*
No	39	52	35	49
Yes:	61	48	65	51
One	36	27	36	30
Two	15	12	16	11
Three or more	10	9	13	10
Where:				
Great Britain	57	72	57	76
Ireland, Channel Islands	4	4	4	3
Mediterranean	21	13	20	9
Other Europe	12	7	13	7
Other abroad	6	4	6	5
	100	100	100	100

In recent years, the elderly have been urged to sustain or improve their health through greater participation in social activities that take the form of physical action, and that usually, but not always, involve others. The Government's General Household Survey carried out throughout 1983 included interviews with 2200 men aged 60 or more and 3088 women of the same age, and asked them about their participation in both outdoor and indoor 'sports, games and physical activities'; only two of these (walking and jogging) did not obviously involve other people simultaneously. In Table 4.2, the results for Great Britain are shown separately for men and women; and for each sex there are comparisons between the pre-elderly (aged 45–59), the younger elderly (aged 60–69) and the older elderly (aged 70 or more).

Table 4.2   Sports, games and physical activities: participation rates in the 4 weeks before the interview (%). Source: *General Household Survey 1983*, p. 203 (HMSO, London, 1986).

(a)   Men

	Age		
	45–59	*60–69*	*70+*
Outdoor			
Walking, 2 miles or more	21	22	13
Football	1	×	0
Golf	5	5	2
Fishing	4	1	×
Swimming (excluding public pools)	3	1	×
Athletics (including jogging)	1	×	0
Cycling	1	1	1
Bowls	2	2	2
Tennis	1	×	×
Cricket	×	×	×
Camping/caravanning	1	1	×
At least one activity (includes some not listed)			
Excluding walking	18	12	6
Including walking	34	31	18
Indoor			
Snooker/billiards, pool	10	5	2
Darts	8	3	1
Swimming	4	2	1
Squash	1	×	0
Badminton	1	×	×
Table tennis	1	×	×
Bowls/tenpin	1	2	2
Gymnastics/athletics	×	×	0
At least one activity (includes some not listed)	22	11	5

(b) Women

	Age		
	45–59	60–69	70+
Outdoor			
Walking, 2 miles or more	20	17	6
Swimming (excluding public pools)	2	1	×
Cycling	1	1	×
Horse riding	×	×	0
Athletics (including jogging)	×	0	0
At least one activity (includes some not listed)			
Excluding walking	8	4	1
Including walking	25	20	7
Indoor			
Swimming	4	3	×
Keep fit/yoga	4	2	1
Darts	3	1	×
Snooker/billiards/pool	1	×	0
Badminton	1	×	0
Squash	×	0	0
At least one activity (includes some not listed)	11	7	2

× = less than 0.5.

Apart from taking a walk of two miles or more, less than one man in five in the pre-elderly years takes part in any outdoor sport, game or physical activity in the average four-week period; even the most extensively patronised of these (golf) occupied only 5 per cent of men. And even walking at least two miles was an achievement recorded by little more than one in five of these pre-elderly men.

Among men in their 60s, walking and golf maintained their relative popularity, but all other outdoor activities of the kind dealt with in the survey were practically abandoned. And among the older elderly these two favourites occupied the time, skill and muscles of scarcely a handful of men aged 70 or more. There is, of course, a substantial loss of muscle strength with advancing age, but it would seem that a fair bit of this loss is simply the result of inactivity among men in their 50s and 60s.

The indoor 'sports, games and physical activities' of men are not likely, given their present form and prevalence, to be of the kind that would replace this lack of outdoor activity. Among pre-elderly men, over a four-week period, four out of every five engaged in none of them; the two most popular indoor activities — snooker and darts — were recorded by 10 per cent and 8 per cent, respectively, of all these men.

Among the younger elderly, the relative indulgence in even these two favourites was halved; among the older elderly, only a very thin scattering of eccentrics claimed that they indulged in any form of indoor activity that could come within the description of 'sports, games and physical activities'. During the daytime and evening, some of the main uses they made of their time were watching television ($3\frac{1}{2}$ hours), listening to the radio ($1\frac{1}{2}$ hours) and 'just resting/taking a nap' ($2\frac{1}{4}$ hours).

Among women in all three age bands, the levels of participation in both outdoor and indoor 'sports, games and physical activities' were usually very much lower than among men. Among those aged 70 or more, for example, even when a walk of two miles or more is included, only 7 per cent of women, as compared with 18 per cent of men, participated in outdoor activities. Participation rates by women in indoor activities, however, at least matched those of men in two of the listed activities: swimming and keep fit/yoga classes. But even here claims by elderly women were extremely low – less than 2 per cent of all women aged 60 or more took part in either of these activities during the average four-week period.

EDUCATION AND THE ELDERLY

These figures, for both elderly men and women, are all the more remarkable in the light of the amount of advice given to them by the non-elderly to keep active and take exercise. Health courses and talks for the elderly have been provided by quangoes, voluntary organisations, academic bodies, etc., in campaigns to promote 'health through activity'. So far, little research has been carried out to measure the reception received by these courses and talks, and why, so often, the reception has been relatively poor.

One such study has recently been carried out by Kathy Meade among 187 pensioners who had attended courses, 19 lecturers who had given the talks and 14 organisers of health courses (Meade, 1986). Of the pensioners, 90 per cent were women, 71 per cent lived alone, 67 per cent had left school by the age of 14, and, most remarkable of all, 64 per cent described themselves as working-class — remarkable because, in Britain and all other countries, a majority of the elderly who attend education courses are almost invariably middle-class.

Some of the findings derived from the answers of the pensioners throw a good deal of light on why the simple message 'be active, be healthy' has not affected the lives of many elderly people. For example, the pensioners were shown six possible reasons why they might have attended, and were asked to indicate which three were most important for them. (The average pensioner provided only 2.8 answers.) Two of the main positive answers were:

53 per cent — 'I wanted to make new friends'.

22 per cent — 'I didn't have anyone to talk to about my health worries'.

Thus, three-quarters were seeking companionship. But the main reason given by 63 per cent of students indicated that they were looking for an escape from boredom — 'I wanted to go to something that wasn't only bingo and chat'. Only 53 per cent of the pensioners used one of the three possible reasons that could be regarded as directly related to the organisers', and lecturers', aims — that is, they 'voted' for the statement, 'I wanted to find out what I could do to keep myself healthy'.

From the answers to questions put to pensioners about the structure and organisation of health education for the elderly, the author concluded that important conditions for communication success, as distinct from companionship success, were:

- Pensioners need to be involved in planning the content of their courses, both in general terms and with regard to individual topics.
- Speakers should be 'briefed' carefully about the interests and needs of the particular group they will be working with.
- Individual sessions should include time for 'private chats' with the speakers afterwards.
- Good teaching aids and leaflets for the pensioners to take home need to be sought out or developed.
- If the group is large, ways of dividing into smaller discussion groups need to be explored (Meade, 1986, p. 24). Nearly half (47 per cent) of the pensioners indicated that they preferred to be taught in classes that contained fewer than 15 pupils (Meade, 1986, p. 14).

When they were asked about the benefits they had derived from the courses they had attended, over half said they had 'continued to meet with new friends they had made' — a proportion well ahead of the 40 per cent who said that they now 'did more exercises at home' even when account is taken of the fact that, of this 40 per cent, nearly three-quarters said they had also attended a special session on 'keeping fit and healthy'.

EXPENDITURE ON LEISURE

In 1985 the average UK household spent £26 in the average week on leisure items; slightly over 70 per cent of this was accounted for by just 4 of the 15 listed forms of leisure: alcoholic drink consumed in pubs and clubs, etc.; holidays; TV licences, cassettes and musical instruments; and meals out. Slightly over 1 per cent went on what might be described (sometimes generously) as cultural leisure activities — that is, charges for admission to theatres, concerts and opera houses, and hobbies.

In the average household where the head was of pensionable age, average weekly expenditure on all the listed forms of entertainment in Table 4.3 was £13, or half that spent by the average UK household. Expenditure on the four items that absorbed over 70 per cent of the average household's expenditure accounted for 65 per cent of the total leisure expenditure of elderly households. Spending by the latter on cultural leisure activities was slightly less than 1 per cent of the total. Thus, it would appear that, among the elderly, expenditure *per head* on leisure goods and services is approximately the same as for the average family in the UK, and that the spending patterns of the two groups are much the same.

There is among elderly people at least as much inequality of income as there is among the non-elderly; and since participation in many leisure activities involves spending money, it is important to distinguish in a social audit of the elderly between the 'aged poor' (that is, those mainly dependent for their income on the State pension) and the 'aged affluent' (that is, those whose State pensions are usually supplemented by an occupational pension and income from their savings and investments). The Government's annual Family Expenditure Survey makes this possible by reporting on four types of households headed by a retired person:

- One person mainly dependent on a State pension; 83 per cent are women (7 per cent of all households).
- Other one-person households; 76 per cent are women (6 per cent of all households).
- Two-person households (one man and one woman) mainly dependent on State pensions (4 per cent of all households).
- Other such two-person households headed by a retired person (6 per cent of all households).

Between them these four types of retired households contain over 90 per cent of all retired persons who are not institutionalised.

Table 4.4 shows how much in 1984 each of these four types of retired household spent on various leisure goods and services. It shows that expenditure on the listed leisure goods and services is highly income-elastic; that is, in both types of elderly household (one-person and two-person) expenditure on these goods and services increases more than it does on all goods and services. This is particularly true of the two-person elderly household, and is accounted for very largely by increased expenditure on transport, holidays and club subscriptions. In other words, with increasing income elderly people turn to commercially provided companionship rather than free companionship from friends and kin.

Table 4.3 Household[a] weekly expenditure on selected leisure items, UK, 1985. Source: *Social Trends*, 17, p. 170 (HMSO, London, 1987)

	(1) All households	(2) Household head over pension age	(2) as % of (1)
Average weekly household expenditure (£) on:			
Alcoholic drink consumed away from home	5.76	1.73	30
Meals consumed out[b]	3.54	1.39	39
Books, papers, magazines, etc.	2.59	1.97	76
Television, radio, musical instruments	4.17	2.16	52
Purchase of materials for home repairs	3.09	2.13	69
Holidays	4.98	3.17	64
Hobbies	0.08	0.03	38
Cinema admissions	0.09	0.02	22
Dance admissions	0.12	0.03	25
Theatre, concert admissions	0.23	0.10	43
Subscription and admission charges to participant sports	0.62	0.18	29
Football match admissions	0.08	0.01	12
Admission to other spectator sports	0.03	0.01	33
Sports goods (excluding clothes)	0.31	0.04	13
Other entertainment	0.30	0.08	27
Total weekly expenditure on above	25.98	13.04	—
Expenditure on above as percentage of all household expenditure	16.0	14.3	50

[a] In 1985 the average household contained 2.56 persons; the size of the average household where the head was of pensionable age or more was 1.43 persons.

[b] Eaten on the premises, excluding State school meals and workplace meals.

Table 4.4 Weekly expenditure (£) by four types of retired household, UK, 1984. Source: *Family Expenditure Survey 1984* (HMSO, London)

Goods and services	One-person household		Two-person household	
	A	B	A	B
Meals bought away from home	0.47	1.32	1.10	2.48
Alcoholic drink	0.99	1.62	2.71	4.63
Reading matter	1.02	1.56	1.70	2.32
Seeds, plants, etc.	0.17	0.52	0.37	0.97
Cars, coach fares, etc.	1.12	5.47	4.70	16.07
Theatres, sporting events, etc.	0.07	0.20	0.10	0.54
TV rental and licence	1.38	1.32	1.75	1.46
Education	–	0.03	–	0.06
Club subscriptions, holidays, etc.	1.51	3.22	1.80	7.31
Total	6.73	15.26	14.23	35.84
As % of all expenditure	17	20	20	28
Total weekly expenditure	38.75	74.73	72.96	128.77
Total weekly expenditure per head	38.75	74.73	36.48	64.38

A, Dependent mainly on a State pension.
B, State pension plus other income.

CONCLUSION

Over the past thirty years there have been many changes that have affected the social lives of elderly people. Some of these have acted to diminish their opportunities for social interaction, while other changes have expanded their opportunities. On the negative side, for example, is the fact that more people are living alone. A national survey carried out in 1959 by Research Services Limited, including 1340 people aged 65 or more, showed that only 11 per cent of men and 33 per cent of women in this age group were living alone; by 1985, however, these proportions had risen to 20 per cent and 47 per cent, respectively.

This trend towards isolation was fortified by the fact that the parents of today's elderly provided them with comparatively few healthy brothers and sisters: one-quarter of those aged 65 years or more are without even one surviving brother or sister, and those who have living siblings rarely see them. In a recent survey of elderly people, one-half of those with living siblings said that they had seen one of them either once a year or even less frequently (Abrams, 1980). Again, in 1959 10 per cent of all those aged 65 or more lived in households that contained children under the age of 15; by 1985 the comparable proportion had fallen to 2 per cent.

These contractions in contact with 'primary' social groups have been accompanied by still another loss of touch among the elderly. In 1959 a quarter of all elderly men were in full-time jobs and thus in everyday contact with workmates; by 1985 only a handful of men — less than 2 per cent — were in this position.

On the positive side, however, technology and higher real incomes have over the same period provided the elderly with new opportunities for social contact. Thirty years ago only 9 per cent of elderly people had a telephone; today the proportion is 75 per cent. Over the same period the proportion of elderly households with a car has risen from 16 per cent to 40 per cent. Over a million people of pensionable age have a Senior Citizens' Rail Card, and many more have bus transport that is either free or else available at greatly reduced fares. The five million elderly who take at least one holiday a year are sufficient in numbers and monetary resources to make it worth while for many travel and tourist agents to provide specialised holidays for them.

Increasingly, the social problem for the elderly is not isolation but lack of appreciation and boredom. Recent surveys have shown that, when interviewed, both the elderly living with others and those living alone initially express satisfaction with the local opportunities for social contact. On further probing, however, it emerges that a sizeable majority among both groups say that in the past few weeks there has been no single occasion when anyone has ever complimented them on something they had done either for themselves or for the community. In further questioning many of these people claimed that they found their lives boring. Clearly, they had not achieved that sense of 'becoming a member of the human community' to which Freud, writing over sixty years ago, attached such importance as a basic condition for happiness.

Perhaps this lack accounts for the attraction of sheltered housing and retirement villages among so many of the elderly. Certainly, it is true that those who can afford to do so tend to move to areas where they are among other elderly people. And those who participate in services provided for the elderly, such as lectures and educational courses, attach great importance to playing a substantial role in shaping the content and organisation of these activities.

REFERENCES

Abrams, M. (1978). *Beyond Three Score and Ten* (A first report on a survey of the elderly), pp. 49–53. Age Concern England, Mitcham
Abrams, M. (1981). *People in Their Late Sixties*, pp. 16–18. Age Concern England, Mitcham

Freud, S. (1973). *Civilisation and its Discontents*, pp. 13, 14. Hogarth Press, London [German Edition, 1970]

Meade, K. (1986). *Challenging the Myths: A Review of Pensioners' Health Courses and Talks*. Health Education Council

5

Geriatric Medicine Today

Michael Hall

INTRODUCTION

The World Health Organization (WHO) defines health as a state of physical, mental and social well-being. Perhaps more than any other hospital-based discipline, geriatric medicine tries to honour this concept. The British Geriatrics Society (BGS) has defined geriatric medicine as 'that branch of general medicine concerned with the clinical, rehabilitative, social and preventive aspects of illness and health in the elderly'. Within this definition, the term 'general medicine' refers to general (internal) medicine in its widest sense, covering all the specialist disciplines such as neurology, cardiology, gastroenterology, etc., while the word 'clinical' covers both physical and mental aspects. This definition expands the WHO definition of health, relates directly to the elderly and places an onus on the hospital-based geriatric medical service to become involved not only in the social aspects of illness, but also in health and the prevention of illness, implying thereby the promotion of health.

The definition raises the question, 'Who are the elderly?' Generally speaking, they have usually been considered as synonymous with the retired — i.e. women over 60 years and men over 65 years. To so define them raises obvious problems. This and other considerations have caused Isaacs (1982) to redefine both the content and the organisation of geriatric medicine. The content comprises the problems of diagnosis, assessment and treatment of illness in older people, usually over 75 years; and the epidemiology of disease in later life. The organisation means providing 'the many forms of medical and social care necessary for the well-being of ill old people, in such a way as to offer choice to the consumer and maximum effectiveness to the provider'.

While this re-definition omits specific mention of health promotion and illness prevention, it stresses the need to provide 'the many forms of medical and social care necessary for the well-being . . . '. The promotion of well-being and the prevention of further disablement in the frail and ageing

65

person can obviously be included among 'the many forms of . . . care'. This re-definition also points out that most of the clientele are aged over 75 years, thereby suggesting the need for an age-defined specialty similar to paediatrics, rather than a specialty which caters for those older people who are likely to benefit most from its ministrations.

THE ORGANISATION OF GERIATRIC MEDICINE

During the past twenty years there has been considerable debate as to the form of the specialty and the role that it should play in the management of illness in older people. Viewpoints have been diverse, ranging from abolition of the specialty (Leonard, 1976) to the provision of a total hospital service for those aged 65 years or more (O'Brien *et al.*, 1973). Support for the specialty has come from within itself via the BGS (Howell, 1974) and from outside via various Department of Health and Social Security (DHSS) Communications, particularly DS 329/71 and the consultative paper on the 'Future pattern of hospital provision in England' (1980); and reports of working parties set up by the Royal Colleges (London, 1977; Edinburgh, 1963 and 1970), as well as the British Medical Association (1949, 1976, 1986).

As a result of these documents, there is no doubt that the specialty is firmly established on a par with other medical specialties and that at least 3 beds per 1000 population aged over 65 years should be available for it in the district general hospital (DGH) (though this figure has not yet been achieved in all districts).

Local district organisation is variable and to a large extent depends on the resources available in the district, the personalities of the physicians in the various specialties and the demands which are likely to be made on the service. In the main, most district geriatric services are so organised that they follow one of two patterns, though in some cases the patterns are modified. These types of service are either 'age-related' or 'integrated'. Before describing the operation of these in greater detail, a brief historical review of the development of geriatric medicine is justified.

HISTORICAL DEVELOPMENT

The early development of the medical care of the elderly by Dr Marjory Warren at the West Middlesex Hospital, Mr Lionel Cosin at Orsett Hospital, Essex, and Drs Eric Brooke and Cooksey at St. Helier Hospital, Carshalton, has been well described by Howell (1974). Williamson (1979) suggests that this was the first phase in development, recognising the importance of full accurate assessment of the individual's physical, mental and social needs before making management decisions; the importance of an appropriate therapeutic environment; and the need to educate doctors and others with regard to the medical problems of old age.

The second phase developed from this, recognising that it was important for the hospital-based doctor to play a part in community care by pre-admission home assessment visiting, thereby educating general practitioners and preventing many admissions; encouraging the development of better community services and liaison with local authorities; and developing day hospitals.

Williamson goes on to suggest that the third phase was the development of preventive geriatric care, beginning with the work of Anderson and Cowan at the Rutherglen Clinic, followed by his own Edinburgh studies on 'unreported needs' (Williamson *et al.*, 1964) and culminating in the setting up of the David Cargill Chair of Geriatric Medicine in the University of Glasgow in 1965. One might perhaps add also the Kilsyth studies organised by this new university department, and finish the phase with the establishment of the first two English Chairs of Geriatric Medicine at Southampton and Manchester in 1970. The first of these was an inaugural Chair in a new medical school; the second, in an expanding medical school, in the University Hospital of South Manchester. The importance of geriatric medicine as a subject to be taught in the undergraduate curriculum was thereby established.

Williamson then suggested that phase IV was with us in 1979 and that we needed to decide whether to abandon the specialty, to opt for an age-related specialty or to foster integration with the rest of medicine while preserving the gains already made. Since the first option was impracticable, we have been left with the second and third.

THE 'AGE-RELATED' SERVICE

The case for an age-related service has been well argued by Horrocks (1982). In this service all patients above a certain age are admitted direct to a bed in the Department of Geriatric Medicine. The age level at which this happens will depend on the resources available to the Department of Geriatric Medicine in the DGH, the demography of the population served and the agreement of colleagues in general medicine. When this type of service is provided, the age aimed at is usually around 75 years, since many observers have suggested that it is above this age that the greatest amount of ill-health and chronic illness exists (Bennett *et al.*, 1970; Evans *et al.*, 1971; McArdle *et al.*, 1975; Hunt, 1978). Some services, however, have the resources to operate a service for all over 65 years (O'Brien *et al.*, 1973; Pathy, 1982), while others with lesser resources have opted for a higher age (Horrocks, 1982).

The advantages of an age-related service may be listed as follows:

- Creation of a specialist department in which older patients are welcome and in which medical skills appropriate to need are immediately available.
- Creation of a therapeutic environment which preserves as well as restores functional independence.
- Negative aspects such as incontinence and mental disturbance are accepted as normal and probably reversible concomitants of illness and not barriers to treatment.
- Generally, a better understanding of the physiological and pathological aspects of ageing.

These are, of course, all prerequisite attitudes and requirements for the management of illness in the elderly, and should be found in any acute ward that admits old people as acute medical emergencies. Other advantages include:

- An operational policy understood by GPs and hospital staff.
- No demarcation disputes with regard to placement of patients.
- An active unit with high turnover is created.
- Recruitment of all grades results from improved staff morale.
- Early referral can be encouraged and long-term institutionalisation may thereby be prevented.

There is no doubt that an age-related service is attractive to many doctors practising geriatric medicine. Criticism that a separate over-75-years age-defined specialty might perpetuate or create a second-class specialty for the aged has not been justified. A more pertinent criticism is that it creates a hospital-based specialty and there is need for geriatric medicine to be highly community-orientated (Williamson, 1979). However, there is no reason why an over-75-year age-defined specialty should not also be community-orientated towards this age group as well as take a specialist interest in those aged 65–74 years who may require the special services that geriatric medicine can provide.

THE 'INTEGRATED' SERVICE

The Royal College of Physicians (London) Working Party on the Care of the Elderly (1977) supported the concept of a service which was integrated closely with general (internal) medicine and proposed that, where appropriate, physicians with an interest in the care of the elderly should be appointed to work alongside physicians with an interest in other specialties.

Thereby geriatric medicine would be closely integrated with hospital general (internal) medical specialties.

The concept of the physician with a major interest in geriatric medicine probably had its origins in Newcastle Regional Hospital Board, which, in the 1960s, advertised the post of consultant physician/geriatrician to develop hospital-based health care services for the elderly. In the autumn of 1962 I was appointed to such a post in Newcastle upon Tyne, to participate in the work of an acute general medical firm and to run the geriatric service; the general medical commitment amounted to three sessions per week and the geriatric medicine commitment to eight sessions. The work involved sharing a medical firm of 40 beds, a 1 in 4 'on-take' commitment and total control of over 350 geriatric beds, of which over 100 were in the DGH. This meant that acutely ill elderly could be admitted to a general medical bed and cared for with the help of the medical firm's junior medical staff, while patients more suitable for 'geriatric medical care' could be managed in the geriatric beds with assistance from Geriatric medical staff.

From this initial base developed the Newcastle Service, which has been well described by Evans (1983), while it has been adapted to fit services in Oxford, London and elsewhere.

THE GERIATRIC PATIENT

The word 'geriatric' has so frequently been used in a pejorative sense that it tends to become synonymous with the witless, incapable, frail elderly pictured in Shakespeare as ' . . . sans everything'. This is, of course, far from being the case, though it will include those whom Isaacs (1974) has described in his classic thesis on *Survival of the Unfittest*. In the case of the agreed 'age-defined' specialty, definition is easy, since it will apply to everyone over the 'cut-off' age. This can mean that very fit and alert people regarding themselves as 'young' will be admitted to geriatric wards. While the treatment that they will receive will be appropriate to their need and age, it may not always be appropriate to themselves or their relatives. One meets here the attitudinal bigotry of ageism (Butler, 1969). The integrated system of care may avoid this difficulty, since the expertise of the geriatrician will be available for those elderly admitted to the acute general medical ward, while the reverse will be true for patients in the geriatric wards.

As a result of experience with the Newcastle system, an attempt was made to define the patient who is more suitably treated in the geriatric medical wards (Hall, 1974). This flow diagram is reproduced for in-patients and out-patients in Figures 5.1 and 5.2. As can be seen, this suggests an age-defined cut-off of 85 years, with younger defined groups being streamed according to their disability. In fact, this streaming exactly mirrors the system which was agreed between the physicians and geriatricians in

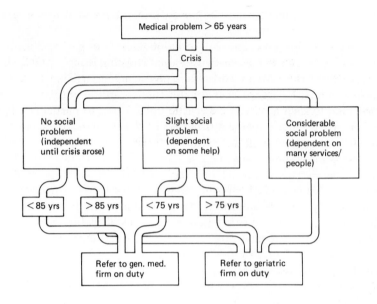

Figure 5.1   In-patient flow diagram

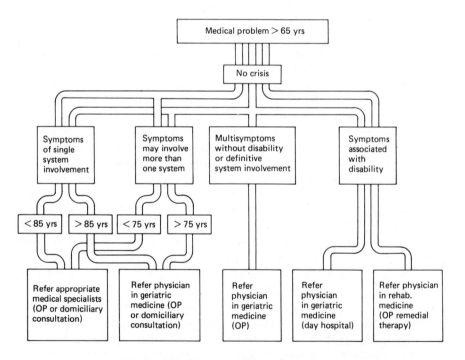

Figure 5.2   Out-patient flow diagram

Southampton when more geriatric beds became available in the DGH in 1982. This arrangement actually arose by chance because it was felt that the geriatric medical resources would only be able to cope with the emergency admissions of those aged 85 years, in addition to the acute admission load of dependent elderly they already carried, only 2 beds per 1000 elderly being available in the DGH. It is interesting, therefore, that an analysis by Nye (1985) of 100 acute random admissions aged 75–84 years to the acute general medical wards compared with a similar number of admissions to the geriatric wards confirmed the greater dependency of the geriatric medical admissions (Figure 5.3).

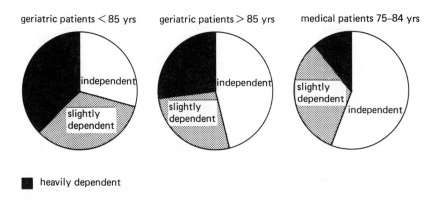

geriatric patients < 85 yrs   geriatric patients > 85 yrs   medical patients 75–84 yrs

heavily dependent

Figure 5.3   Dependency of acute admission to geriatric and general medical beds

PATTERNS OF PROVISION

As has already been emphasised, the resources available to the geriatric medical service will inevitably affect the type of hospital service it can offer. The DHSS norm is that 10 beds per 1000 elderly population should be devoted to the specialty and that at least 3 of these beds should be in the DGH. The reasons for this norm are enshrouded in the mists of time, and more recently Slattery and Bourne (1979) have argued that a figure of 8 beds per 1000 elderly is more realistic.

Figure 5.4 shows the considerable range of beds available to geriatric medicine in 161 districts in England and Wales. The siting of these beds will also influence the type of service that can be provided. Pathy (1982) suggests that if a unit is to have a high turnover, then the majority of its beds need to be in the DGH. Woodford-Williams (1982) states that a unit turning over less than 5 patients per bed (bed factor of 5) per annum needs to be reviewed. Hospital in-patient enquiry (HIPE) figures for 1978 showed a bed factor of only 4.8 for geriatric medicine. In Hull (Bagnall *et al.*, 1977) the

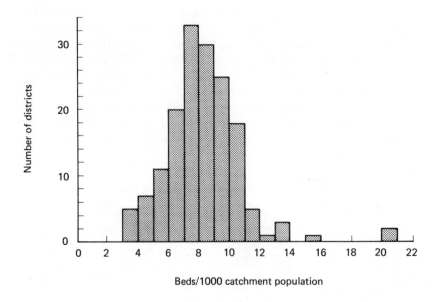

Figure 5.4   Available beds per consultant physician in geriatrics, 1981 (161 districts)

factor was 9. Figure 5.5 shows that the average length of stay varied considerably and it is unlikely that districts with a long average length of stay will achieve the turnover which Woodford-Williams suggests. Turnover, however, is only one measure of the success of a unit. It will not necessarily measure efficacy of treatment and the efficiency and effectiveness of a geriatric service may be better assessed by using a variety of performance indicators.

Efficiency will depend not only on the organisation and placement of beds, but also on staffing. It is generally accepted that the three clinical components of a service will be acute (often called acute assessment), rehabilitation and long-stay. In 1982 a postal questionnaire was sent to consultants in the 289 Geriatric Departments in the United Kingdom to ascertain the type of practice undertaken (Brocklehurst and Andrews, 1985). Combined acute and rehabilitation with separate long-stay (AR/L) was the commonest mix (37.5 per cent), with separate facilities (A/R/L) accounting for 24.4 per cent and combined facilities (ARL) for 21.2 per cent. The fourth alternative, separate acute with combined rehabilitation and long-stay (A/RL), accounted for only 7.5 per cent. The remaining units (9.3 per cent) had variable patterns, and some 2.3 per cent had no acute beds. Total beds per 1000 over-65-years population varied from 9.55 in AR/L to 7.94 in A/RL; beds per consultant varied from 140.88 in AR/L to 120.30 in ARL; the bed factor varied from 3.93 in A/RL to 5.21 in A/R/L, which also had the highest rate of discharges per head of population (42.63).

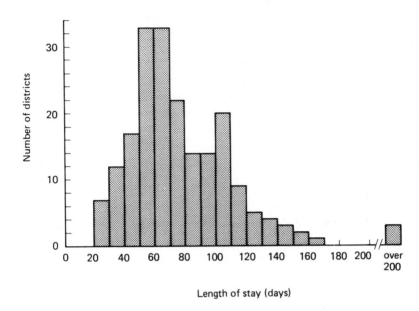

Figure 5.5 Length of stay in geriatrics, 1981 (200 districts)

While the results of this survey are interesting, in that they suggest that separate facilities (A/R/L) may produce marginally better results, we have little information concerning the effect of other factors such as collaboration with other medical services (including primary medical care), Social Services provision, housing provision, and the voluntary and private agencies.

COLLABORATION WITH OTHER SPECIALTIES

Many older people are catered for by other specialties and there is no need for the geriatric medical specialty to become involved in their care. In some cases the help of other specialties may be sought. This, of course, applies particularly to the surgical specialties, since many admissions have conditions which may respond to the appropriate treatment. It is now accepted that age is no bar to even major surgical procedures, so that cardiac surgery and major joint replacement are now commonplace. The special senses deteriorate with age, and sensory deprivation may accentuate loneliness and underlie psychiatric illness. Surveys have shown that almost a third of the over-65s are hard of hearing; therefore a good audiology service is important. Hearing therapists are now becoming a regular part of the therapeutic team. Similarly, the ophthalmic surgeon and the optician have important roles to play in the maintenance of vision.

With some specialties close liaison has been developed, since many patients have common problems. With orthopaedic surgery common wards and services were established in Hastings (Irvine, 1982) and this model has been adopted by or adapted in many centres (Irvine and Strouthidis, 1977).

Incontinence is common, occurring in 18 per cent of women and 7 per cent of men over 65 years (Vetter, 1981). The importance of the condition was recognised long ago by Brocklehurst (1951), and the stimulus of his research (Brocklehurst and Dillane, 1966a,b; 1967a,b) has led to the development of incontinence clinics and the positive promotion of continence, with the appointment in some districts of advisory nurses. Close links, therefore, must be developed between geriatric medicine specialists and their colleagues in urology, gynaecology and medical physics, in order to promote research and develop better methods of management and treatment. Indeed, the provision of a district continence advisor, urodynamic investigation unit and incontinence laundry service are all included in the checklist provided by Horrocks (1986) as components of a comprehensive district health service for elderly people.

PSYCHIATRIC SERVICES FOR THE ELDERLY

The problems of mental health in old age were first highlighted by Roth (1955), and community-orientated psychiatric services for the elderly were developed in the late 1950s and early 1960s (MacMillan, 1960; Robinson, 1965). It soon became apparent that patients referred had much in common with those referred to geriatric medicine (Kidd, 1962). The case for close collaboration between geriatric medicine and psychiatry was proposed in 1966 (Kay *et al.*). This paper emphasised that one of the key concepts in modern geriatric care was integration of services 'with a proper balance between hospital and community care'. It also suggested the creation of a comprehensive psychogeriatric assessment unit (PGAU) which would be situated in the DGH, staffed by physicians and psychiatrists, supported by out-patient and day hospital facilities, and closely integrated with the general practitioner service and local authority Social Service departments.

In 1970 the DHSS Circular HM (70) 11 supported the promotion of psychogeriatric units to facilitate collaboration between psychiatrists, geriatricians and social workers. However, as Godber (1978) pointed out, the joint PGAU recommended was small (10–20 beds per 250 000 population) and the potential case load is extremely large. Consequently, to operate efficiently, rapid turnover of patients in this unit was essential, and if beds became 'blocked', the unit failed. However, where resources were adequate and when operational policies could be agreed between all agencies, such units operated successfully (Donovan *et al.*, 1971).

Nevertheless, conflict still exists, and in many districts the overall service to the elderly patient is deficient. Godber (1978) has suggested that the way forward is the merging of the two specialties of geriatric psychiatry and geriatric medicine into a single administrative unit. This is a bold and imaginative concept. However, it is not likely to be achieved overnight, although the creation of the Department of Health Care of the Elderly at Nottingham is pointing the way, the organisation and style of psychogeriatric services has been clearly described (Arie and Jolley, 1982), and the Standing Joint Committee of the British Geriatrics Society and the Royal College of Psychiatrists has agreed guidelines on liaison (Royal College of Psychiatrists, 1979).

It is tragic that so much time and energy has had to be spent establishing geriatric medicine as a specialty in its own right when, given appropriate resources, a much more comprehensive service involving all relevant agencies might now be in existence, so meeting the criteria necessary to meet 'the rising tide' (NHSHAS, 1982).

REHABILITATION

Rehabilitation, sometimes called re-enablement, is an essential component of any geriatric service. Ideally beds should be on the same site as the District Rehabilitation Department and a close liaison needs to be developed with rehabilitation medicine. Physiotherapists and occupational therapists, speech therapists and hearing therapists are all important members of the multidisciplinary team which is necessary to enable the elderly patient to regain function and return to the community. Impaired ability is a common reason for people to be referred to the Geriatric Department. Time is not on the side of the elderly patient, and, consequently, accurate multidisciplinary assessment and expeditious treatment of disability are essential. The construction of a management plan, the setting of realistic goals, and the close monitoring of progress are essential.

Geriatric rehabilitation services are often divided into fast/medium- and slow-stream sections, the fast stream being situated in the DGH, the slow stream in less expensive longer-stay accommodation. Patients requiring rehabilitation should be admitted initially to fast/medium-stream beds unless their needs have previously been assessed, in which case admission to a slow-stream bed may be appropriate. Patients may be admitted direct from home or transferred from an acute ward. Resources in the DGH are expensive, and patients needing rehabilitation should be transferred from acute beds as soon as possible, and if their progress is then slow, transferred to a slow-stream bed.

Perhaps the most important aspect of rehabilitation services for the elderly is to ensure that they work. Rosenberg and his colleagues (1986) report that the institution of a new record system for rehabilitation improved the discharge rate and, therefore, turnover in a rehabilitation hospital. It is likely that this was the direct result of better and clearer documentation of the patient's abilities, management and achievements, linked to discharge plans made and recorded early in the admission. The creation of specialist areas within the rehabilitation service such as 'stroke' ward or unit may have the same effect of expediting discharge (Garraway *et al.*, 1980).

Whatever the system adopted, additional supportive community services such as the day hospital, 'Stroke' Clubs, domiciliary physiotherapy, occupational therapy, speech therapy and hearing therapy may enable the elderly patient to be discharged earlier and maintain his or her function at an optimal level.

THE DAY HOSPITAL

The concept of 'day hospitals' originated in psychiatry in the 1930s and the first purpose-designed geriatric day hospital was built at Cowley Road, Oxford, under the direction of Lionel Cosin in the 1950s. Since then it has become an integral part of the hospital-based geriatric medical and psychiatric service. It has been defined as a hospital ward from which the patients return home to sleep each night. Thereby it provides treatment on a daily basis to patients, enabling them to remain in their own homes. Its functions can be investigative, curative and rehabilitative as well as maintaining an individual's function at an optimal level. It may, therefore, have a social role in addition to its undoubted therapeutic role.

Doubt, however, still exists with regard to many aspects of the day hospital. How large should it be? Martin and Millard (1976) suggest not more than 18 places. How many day hospital places are necessary in a district? The DHSS norm is 2 places per 1000 aged 65 years or more for medical patients and 2–3 places per 1000 aged 65 years or more for psychiatric patients. Few, if any, districts will have achieved these figures.

Reviews and studies with regard to day hospitals and their function (Brocklehurst, 1970; Arie, 1975; Martin and Millard, 1978; Irvine, 1980; Brocklehurst and Tucker, 1980; Tucker, 1982) have not completely answered these and the many other questions with regard to the value and place of the day hospital in the hospital geriatric service.

LONG-TERM CARE

A proportion of the total number of beds allocated to geriatric medicine in each health district are devoted to the care of patients who have proved irremediable and consequently require permanent long-term care. The siting of these beds varies. In some units patients remain in the ward to which they were originally admitted, but in most cases they are moved to a specific long-stay ward, now sometimes called a continuing care ward, which may be situated in a peripheral hospital. This hospital will, if possible, be nearer to the patient's own home, thereby making it easier for relatives to visit. However, in many districts these wards are in old 'Poor Law' hospitals or designated geriatric hospitals. To provide care of good quality in such institutions can be difficult. This has been recognised, and steps have been taken in many places to improve the quality of life for old people placed in such hospitals. It has also been suggested that smaller nursing units may provide a more 'homely' atmosphere, and three experimental nursing homes have been set up by the DHSS. Publications such as James Elliott's *Living in Hospitals*, published by the King Edward's Hospital Fund for London (1975), and Denham's excellent book *Care of the Long-stay Elderly Patient* have done much to stimulate discussion and bring about improvements in care in this difficult area of geriatric medicine.

Many 'long-stay units' also operate 'respite care beds' and participate in long-term rehabilitation. This means that they have a mixed function, and because they have a changing clientele, nursing staff are easier to obtain. These units are ideally suited to cater for these categories of patient. Their more 'homely atmosphere' and more personalised treatment programmes will often stimulate further recovery, which can then be built on.

RESPITE CARE

'Respite care' may be given to appropiate patients to give their carers relief on either a regular or an irregular basis. On a regular basis, it has become an adaptation of the 'six weeks in; six weeks out' scheme (De Largy, 1957). In many cases the 'in' period has been shortened to two weeks, so that the scheme becomes one of 'two weeks in; six (or sometimes four) weeks out'. In this way, by sharing the care of the elderly dependent patient, carers can be relieved to some extent of their burden of care, the patient maintained at an optimal level of function and often improved, and a permanent long-term admission prevented, so that one bed can be used on a rotational basis to cater for three or even four patients.

'Respite' or 'relief' or 'holiday' admissions have, however, been criticised in that they may be detrimental to the patient. It is generally accepted that there is a potential risk of death occurring when a frail, dependent, ill elderly patient is transferred from one hospital to another. Rai *et al.* (1986) have recently reported an increased death rate among 'holiday' admissions, attributing this to the admission. This, however, has not been the experience of others, though all who have operated such schemes will have experienced some deaths within this clientele, as one might expect.

There is no doubt that this group pose an ethical problem. On the one hand, there is the patient who probably wishes to remain at home, often regardless of physical and mental disability; on the other hand, the carer(s), who may have to carry an impossible burden of care. Sanford (1975) has reviewed the burdens which carers find difficult to tolerate. High on this list are disturbed nights, irrational behaviour and faecal incontinence, all of which will cause the most willing carer to give up unless relieved either regularly or 'on demand'. To be successful, 'respite' or 'holiday' admissions need to be carefully planned and the informed consent of the patient and carer(s) needs to be obtained. The medical/nursing team at both ends — i.e. the hospital and the patient's home — need to be involved so that admissions/discharges are planned. Schemes should not operate 'automatically' and patients should not be admitted/discharged because the due date has been reached.

Like many aspects of geriatric medicine (see below), 'respite care' requires a clear operational policy which needs to be adhered to and monitored. In this way the benefits or otherwise of the scheme to both patients and carer(s) can be assessed and modified when and where necessary.

THE COMPREHENSIVE DISTRICT HEALTH SERVICE FOR THE ELDERLY

This chapter has so far outlined the development of the specialty of geriatric medicine and defined its objectives. It has concentrated on the hospital, and little has yet been said about the community other than to mention its importance. Moreover, little has been said about the efficacy of the specialty, and the present chapter would be incomplete without some discussion of this.

Horrocks (1986) has recently presented a model comprehensive district health service for the elderly. This model is based on his personal experience as a Consultant in Geriatric Medicine and as Director of the NHS Health Advisory Service (HAS) for England and Wales in recent years. In this he states that 'no one Health District currently offers the whole range of provision envisaged' in his paper. Horrocks points out that to make good practice more general represents a major need and that existing knowledge must be made more easily available. The HAS maintains an index of good practice and can refer inquirers to it. This is very important, if standards of practice are to be improved. An enormous amount of information already exists, but because much of it is unrecorded, there is a tendency for planners to repeatedly 'reinvent the wheel'. Many excellent schemes, introduced by various entrepreneurs, which would greatly benefit patient care fail largely because they are not adequately assessed, and then either implemented or discarded or rationalised. As Isaacs (1984) states in the introduction to *Innovations in the Care of the Elderly*, it is relatively easy to have a good idea. Implementing it is much harder, for one has to overcome objections from practically everyone concerned with the change, not least from the intended beneficiary. Implementation can only be achieved as a result of considerable planning. The policy underlying the idea needs to be defined, debated and perhaps modified before it is tried out, perhaps initially in the form of a pilot study. Ideas which are imposed without such preliminaries rarely work, and often cause resentment and a general lowering of morale. Finally, the policy, having been implemented, must be monitored and audited and shown to work. This invariably means that it must be measured against a control group or that the study must be planned in such a way that it acts as its own control. Such planned operational research is rare; yet it is essential if we are to make real progress. The appropriate use and best use of resources is an essential rule of good housekeeping. This means efficiency. Yet efficiency must be tempered by humanism. In other words, a comprehensive district health service for the elderly needs to have resources and use them effectively to promote the quality of life for elderly people.

Twenty years ago, Kay and his colleagues (1966) suggested that a service orientated towards preventive care needed five components:

1. An organisation and administrative structure which facilitates integration on a practical level of the various component parts of the service.
2. A scheme of ascertainment of those most likely to need help.
3. A number of lines of defence within the community designed to serve differing needs of old people. These would include domiciliary services, leisure activities and clubs, and continuing education, as well as health resources provided by the general practitioner, community health and hospitals.
4. Hospital in-patient services, available on demand or as part of a planned programme.
5. Provision of long-term accommodation, which would include residential homes and 'sheltered' housing of various kinds.

Horrocks (1986), concentrating more on the provision of a health service, nevertheless stresses the importance of an overall common philosophy and the integration of health and other services for the elderly. He emphasises the importance of 'locality planning', sometimes called 'patch planning', and of accurate information and feedback in the provision of a rational, effective overall service.

PLANNING

If a good comprehensive district health service for the elderly is to exist,
then good planning is essential, for only through planning can the total
resources available be used efficiently and effectively (Klemperer and
McClenahan, 1981). From the hospital viewpoint, the introduction of 'the
Griffiths management structure' could in theory make the provision of such
a service easier. However 'the elderly' are not a homogeneous group: they
have many 'medical' needs which cross many disciplinary boundaries.
Consequently, they have hospital-based needs as well as community health
needs, in addition to needs met by services provided by social services and
housing committees and by voluntary agencies and the private sector.
Horrocks (1986) stresses the value of Joint Consultative Committees and the
role of the Community Health Council in aiding the planning of the use of
resources. However, as far as health is concerned, the needs of the elderly
are unlikely to be met by one unit of management, and the new management
procedures may make collaboration more difficult. The study undertaken by
Southampton University for the DHSS enabled the Health and Social
Services planning in the period 1979–82 to be studied (Wright and Sheldon,
1985). The work of Health Care Planning Teams and the Joint Finance
Executive were examined. Although this research took place before the
most recent reorganisation of the Health Service in April 1982, its findings
should not be ignored, since joint planning still has to take place. Six factors
in particular seemed to be important:

1. Personalities sufficiently high up in their own service to carry authority, who understand joint planning procedures and who can work well
   together.
2. A small group with a consistent membership (ideally less than twelve
   members).
3. Clear agreed operational guidelines between services and members;
   tasks to be set/goals to achieve.
4. Adequate databases from which to operate.
5. Links with other planning levels, representation on other joint/
   internal planning meetings and direct reporting to major decision-
   making/decision-taking bodies.
6. Time for relationships within the group to develop, so that members
   are not defensive about their own services.

To these six factors should be added: representation on the group of each
service/agency concerned with the elderly.
   As a result of this study, such a group has been formed in the Southampton and South-West Hampshire Health Authority District. It has so far

reported on day care and is currently studying long-term care. It is serviced by an administrator from the Health Authority. The membership includes senior social services officers, a consultant geriatrician, a consultant psycho-geriatrician and a general practitioner, a senior representative of community nursing services, officers from District Housing Committees responsible for elderly housing, the Chief Officer of Age Concern (Hampshire), the Secretary of the Hampshire Rest Homes Association and a representative from the Voluntary Housing Association. The group reports at regular intervals to a member group comprising appointed members of the Health Authority and elected members of the local authority Social Services Committee and District Housing Committees. The member group is chaired by the Chairman of the District Health Authority.

It is too early to assess the value of this experiment, but the first signs are encouraging. Similar groups are also beginning to develop in other parts of the United Kingdom.

THE WAY FORWARD

Arie and his colleagues (1985), discussing education and old age psychiatry services, quote Brice Pitt as describing psychogeriatrics 'as belonging to the family of psychiatry, married to geriatrics, and conducting a fairly turbulent affair with social services'. Medical services for the elderly clearly need to be linked to the provision of social services, housing, and the voluntary and private sector.

Wistow (1982) has defined collaboration as the co-ordination of services, often provided by different agencies in the provision of 'continuous' or 'total' care for a particular patient or client. It would appear to operate at two levels. One, 'higher', involves professionals actively working together and helping each other by using their own resources. Activities would involve joint assessment, reciprocal consultation and case conferences. The second, 'lower', level involves professionals being aware of another's activities and taking these into account while carrying out their own. Knowledge and sympathetic understanding of other people's roles and efficient communication channels are essential at both levels.

A study to look at collaboration at the field level between hospital-based and community-based services in the case of elderly mentally infirm people was undertaken by Southampton University on behalf of the DHSS between 1979 and 1982 (Wright *et al.*, 1986). This study concluded that there were only 'pockets' of the higher level of collaboration between disciplinary teams, based on joint assessment of cases, on sharing care and resources.

There was slightly more evidence of collaboration at the lower level, as judged by appropriate exchange of referrals between services and the satisfactory provision of resources. The majority of contacts between services was also at the lower level. Services tended to work in physical and effectual isolation from each other's resources. Most contacts were by letter or telephone, and referrals were on–off requests for assistance at the referrer's initiative and independent of the appropriateness of the request. There were few formal links, and role expectations were frequently misinformed, so that professionals were stereotyped.

Some positive aspects of collaboration, however, did come out of this research.

For instance, with regard to teamwork, it was clear that for teamwork and collaboration to be successful it was necessary, within teams, for there to be: regular team meetings for adequate communication about patient care; understanding between different professions; airing of grievances and resolution of conflict; informal and formal referral/discussion of cases; adequate resources; face-to-face contact of team members; positive motivation towards team work; acceptance of leadership; ability to compromise to fit with overall team goals.

Between teams the most important aspects were: positive motivation towards collaboration; adequate resources to reduce the compensation element of one service 'helping' another while the other was 'overprotective' towards its own resources; formal links; physical proximity and face-to-face contact to promote mutual understanding of roles and resources; agreed policies, particularly in relation to transfer and referral cases, in order to minimise disputes over 'borderline' cases; simplification of administrative structures and boundaries. This latter point is particularly important, since if geographical areas are defined, 'patch planning' can proceed.

A good example of this has been described by Patnaik (1984). In this case, geriatric medical beds have been linked with local authority residential home beds and both local authority and community health services, to provide a service for a defined geographical catchment area. The district was divided into four sectors each containing approximately the same number of elderly, and the resources available to both agencies were thereby shared on an equal basis, to provide a community-orientated service.

Many other examples of collaborative practices have been devised. An excellent scheme for identifying those most likely to need help was described by Munday and Rowe (1979) in relation to general practices in Devon. This scheme, however, like many others, requires continual monitoring and review. Often the administrative backing is not available to keep information systems up to date, and unless this happens, they fail. The same comment applies to computerised systems, although information, if properly coded, may be extracted more easily from these.

There are grounds for optimism. The need for more integration of services has been widely recognised and there is now some evidence of concern to move this from theory to practice. However, a major obstacle remains: as long as budgets remain tied to specific groups and regulations prevent the transfer of funds across organisational boundaries, a truly comprehensive and integrated service will be very difficult, if not impossible, to achieve.

CONCLUSION

This chapter has attempted to look at the overall development of geriatric medicine as a discipline linked to general (internal) medicine, yet operating closely with the psychiatry of old age (psychogeriatrics) and the community services. It has also described in some detail the range of services that now comprise and involve geriatric medicine.

A great deal has been achieved in the forty years since the inception of the NHS, but it is only recently that steps have been taken towards the provision of a truly comprehensive and integrated service for older people. This is where the current challenge lies, and geriatric medicine has a key role to play in the planning as well as the delivery of these services.

REFERENCES

Arie, T. (1975). Day care in geriatric psychiatry. *Gerontol. Clin.*, **17**, 31

Arie, T. D. H. and Jolley, D. J. (1982). Making services work: Organisation and style of psychogeriatric services. In Levy, R. and Post, F. (Eds.), *The Psychiatry of Later Life*, pp. 222–251. Blackwell Scientific, Oxford

Arie, T., Jones, R. and Smith, C. (1985). The educational potential of old age psychiatry services. In Arie, T. (Ed.), *Recent Advances in Psychogeriatrics*, pp. 197–207. Churchill Livingstone, Edinburgh

Bagnall, W. E., Datta, S. R., Knox, J., *et al.* (1977). Geriatric medicine in Hull: a comprehensive service. *Br. Med. J.*, **2**, 102

Bennett, A. E., Garrad, J. and Halil, T. (1970). Chronic disease and disability in the community: a prevalence study. *Br. Med. J.*, **3**, 762

British Medical Association (1949). *The Care and Treatment of the Elderly and Infirm.* BMA, London

British Medical Association (1976). *The Care of the Elderly.* BMA, London

British Medical Association (1986). *All Our Tomorrows: Growing Old in Britain.* Report of its Board of Science and Education (discussion document). BMA, London

Brocklehurst, J. C. (1951). *Incontinence in Old Age.* Livingstone, Edinburgh

Brocklehurst, J. C. (1970). *The Geriatric Day Hospital.* King Edward's Hospital Fund, London

Brocklehurst, J. C. and Andrews, K. (1985). Geriatric medicine. The style of practice. *Age and Ageing*, **14**, 1

Brocklehurst, J. C. and Dillane, J. B. (1966a). Studies of the female bladder in old age. I. Cystometrograms in non-incontinent women. *Gerontol. Clin.*, **8**, 285

Brocklehurst, J. C. and Dillane, J. B. (1966b). Studies of the female bladder in old age. II. Cystometrograms in 100 incontinent women. *Gerontol. Clin.*, **8**, 306

Brocklehurst, J. C. and Dillane, J. B. (1967a). Studies of the female bladder in old age. III. Micturating cystograms in incontinent women. *Gerontol. Clin.*, **9**, 47

Brocklehurst, J. C. and Dillane, J. B. (1967b). Studies of the female bladder in old age. IV. Drug effects in urinary incontinence. *Gerontol. Clin.*, **9**, 182

Brocklehurst, J. C. and Tucker, J. S. (1980). *Progress in Geriatric Day Care*. King Edward's Hospital Fund, London

Butler, R. N. (1969). Age-ism another form of bigotry. *Gerontologist*, **9**, 243

De Largy, J. (1957). Six weeks in: six weeks out. *Lancet*, **1**, 418

Denham, J. J. (Ed.) (1983). *Care of the Long-stay Elderly Patient*. Croom Helm, London

Department of Health and Social Security (1970). *Psychogeriatric Assessment Units* (Health Memorandum (70) 11). HMSO, London

Department of Health and Social Security (1971). *Hospital Geriatric Services*. HMSO, London

Department of Health and Social Security (1980). *Future Pattern of Hospital Provision in England* (consultative paper). HMSO, London

Donovan, J. F., Williams, I. E. I. and Wilson, T. D. (1971). A fully integrated psychogeriatric service. In Kay, D. W. K. and Walk, A. (Eds.), *Recent Developments in Psychogeriatrics*. Royal Medico-Psychological Association, London

Elliot, J. R. (1975) *Living in Hospital*. King Edward's Hospital Fund, London

Evans, G. J., Hodkinson, H. M. and Mezey, A. G. (1971). The elderly sick: who looks after them? *Lancet*, **2**, 539

Evans, J. G. (1983). Integration of geriatric with general medical services in Newcastle. *Lancet*, **1**, 1430

Garraway, W. M., Akhtar, A. J., Hockey, L., *et al.* (1980). Management of acute stroke in the elderly: Follow-up of a controlled trial. *Br. Med. J.*, **2**, 827

Godber, Colin (1978). Conflict and collaboration between geriatric medicine and psychiatry. In Isaacs, B. (Ed.), *Recent Advances in Geriatric Medicine*, Vol. I, pp. 131–142. Churchill Livingstone, Edinburgh

Hall, M. R. P. (1974). Geriatric medicine and its role in the care of the elderly. In Hall, M. R. P. (Ed.), *Aspects of Geriatric Medicine*, pp. 1465–1480. *Medicine*, **25**, 1972–1974 Series

Horrocks, Peter (1982). The case for geriatric medicine as an age-related specialty. In Isaacs, B. (Ed.), *Recent Advances in Geriatric Medicine*, Vol. II, pp. 260–267. Churchill Livingstone, Edinburgh

Horrocks, Peter (1986). The components of a comprehensive District Health Service for elderly people — a personal view. *Age and Ageing*, **15**, 321

Howell, Trevor (1974). Origins of the British Geriatric Society. *Age and Ageing*, **3**, 69

Hunt, A. (1978). *The Elderly at Home*. HMSO, London

Irvine, R. E. (1980). Geriatric day hospitals: Present trends. *Hlth Trends*, **12**, 68

Irvine, R. E. (1982). A geriatric orthopaedic unit. In Coakley, D. (Ed.), *Establishing a Geriatric Service*, pp. 166–180. Croom Helm, London

Irvine, R. E. and Strouthidis, T. M. (1977). Medical care in geriatric orthopaedics. In Devas, M. (Ed.), *Geriatric Orthopaedics*, pp. 11–29. Academic Press, London

Isaacs, B. (1974). *Survival of the Unfittest: Studies of Illness and Death in the Elderly in Glasgow* (Scottish Health Service Study No. 17). Scottish Home and Health Department

Isaacs, B. (1982). Introduction: Geriatric medicine: the state of the nation. In Isaacs, B. (Ed.), *Recent Advances in Geriatric Medicine*, Vol. II. Churchill Livingstone, Edinburgh

Isaacs, B. (1984). Introduction: In Isaacs, B. and Evers, H. (Eds.), *Innovations in the Care of the Elderly*, pp. 1–2. Croom Helm, London

Kay, D. W. K., Roth, M. and Hall, M. R. P. (1966). Special problems of the aged and the organisation of hospital services. *Br. Med. J.*, **2**, 967

Kidd, C. B. (1962). Misplacement of the elderly in hospital. *Br. Med. J.*, **2**, 1491

Klemperer, P. D. and McClenahan, J. W. (1981). Joint strategic planning between Health and Local Authority. *Omega*, **5**, 481

Leonard, J. C. (1976). Can geriatrics survive? *Br. Med. J.*, **2**, 1335

McArdle, C., Wylie, J. C. and Alexander, W. D. (1975). Geriatric patients in an acute medical ward. *Br. Med. J.*, **4**, 568

MacMillan, D. (1960). Preventive geriatrics. *Lancet*, **2**, 1439

Martin, A. and Millard, P. H. (1976). Effect of size on the function of the Day Hospitals; the case for the small unit. *J. Am. Geriat. Soc.*, **24**, 506

Martin, A. and Millard, P. H. (1978). *Day Hospitals for the Elderly — Therapeutic or Social?* St. George's Hospital, London

Munday, M. and Rowe, J. (1979). *Care of the Elderly in Devon*. King Edward's Hospital Fund, London

NHSHAS (National Health Service Health Advisory Service) (1982). *The Rising Tide*. HMSO, London

Nye, Fiona (1985). A Comparison of the Reasons for Admissions of Patients aged 75 Years and over to the Acute Medical Wards, with Those Admitted to the Geriatric Unit in the Southampton General Hospital. University of Southampton, Faculty of Medicine, 4th Year Medical Student Project

O'Brien, T. D., Joshi, D. M. and Warren, E. W. (1973). No apology for geriatrics. *Br. Med. J.*, **4**, 277

Pathy, J. (1982). Operational policies. In Coakley, D. (Ed.), *Establishing a Geriatric Service*, pp. 37–57. Croom Helm, London

Patnaik, B. K. (1984). The therapeutic community at Grantham and Kesteven Hospital. *Action Baseline* (Spring), 22

Rai, G. S., Bielawska, C., Murphy, P. J. and Wright, G. (1986). Hazards for elderly people admitted for respite ('holiday admissions') and social care ('social admissions'). *Br. Med. J.*, **292**, 240

Robinson, R. A. (1965). A psychiatric geriatric unit. In *Psychiatric Disorders in the Aged*, pp. 186–205. World Psychiatric Association Symposium, Geigy

Rosenberg, W., Parkes, J., Jenkins, A., *et al.* (1986). Making a Rehabilitation Hospital for the elderly work. *Hlth Trends*, **18**, 66

Roth, M. (1955). The natural history of mental disorder in old age. *J. Ment. Sci.*, **101**, 281

Royal College of Physicians (Edinburgh) (1963). *Care of the Elderly in Scotland*. No. 22. Royal College of Physicians, Edinburgh

Royal College of Physicians (Edinburgh) (1970). *Care of the Elderly in Scotland*. A Follow-up Report. Royal College of Physicians, Edinburgh

Royal College of Physicians (London) (1977). *Report of the Working Party on Medical Care of the Elderly*. Royal College of Physicians, London

Royal College of Psychiatrists (1979). Guidelines for collaboration between geriatric physicians and psychiatrists in the care of the elderly. *Roy. Coll. Psychiat. Bull.*, November, 168

Sanford, J. R. A. (1975). Tolerance and debility in elderly dependents by supporters at home: its significance for hospital practice. *Br. Med. J.*, **3**, 471

Slattery, M. and Bourne, A. (1979). Norms and recent trends in Geriatrics. *J. Clin. Exp. Gerontol.*, **1**, 79

Tucker, J. S. (1982). The day hospital. In Coakley, D. (Ed.), *Establishing a Geriatric Service*, pp. 58–70. Croom Helm, London

Vetter, N. J., Jones, Dee A. and Victor, Christina R. (1981). Urinary incontinence in the elderly at home. *Lancet*, **1**, 1275

Williamson, J. (1979). Three views of geriatric medicine. 3. Notes on the historical development of geriatric medicine as a medical specialty. *Age and Ageing*, **8**, 144

Williamson, J., Stokoe, I. H., Gray, S., Fisher, M., Smith, A., McGhee, A. and Stephenson, E. (1964). Old people at home: their unreported needs. *Lancet*, **1**, 1117

Wistow, E. (1982). Collaboration between Health and Local Authorities. Why is it necessary? *Soc. Pol. Admin.*, **16**, 44

Woodford-Williams, E. (1982). The efficiency and quality of the service. In Coakley, D. (Ed.), *Establishing a Geriatric Service*, pp. 106–112. Croom Helm, London

Wright, Jenny, Ball, Carolyn and Coleman, Peter (1986). *Collaboration between Hospital and Community Services in the Care of the Elderly Mentally Infirm.* University of Southampton, Departments of Geriatric Medicine and Social Work Studies

Wright, Jennifer and Sheldon, Frances (1985). Health and social services planning. *Soc. Pol. Admin.*, **19**, 258

6

Demographic and Health Trends in the Elderly

Michael Alderson

INTRODUCTION

This chapter sets out information on the demographic changes that have occurred this century in England and Wales, with particular emphasis on aspects related to the elderly. It then considers what is known about the major diseases killing the elderly and trends in these diseases, and reviews other statistics on the health problems of the elderly. The scope is restricted to routine statistics; data are available on mortality from all causes, cancer trends (incidence and survival as well as mortality), diagnoses for hospital in-patients, sample material from three periodic studies on contact in primary medical care, and annual surveys on the general level of disability in the population. Consideration is given to the facilities and support that are utilised in caring for the elderly, and an attempt is made to identify the proportion of the population by age and sex receiving care from the main agencies. Limited material is also available on selected facets of 'behaviour': diet, alcohol consumption and smoking. Consideration of these issues is relevant to the health of the general population and health of the elderly. The final section discusses projections of the elderly population over the coming forty years in the United Kingdom and considers the possible degree of handicap in these elderly.

All the results are based on routinely available data; the primary source of such material is given, though appreciable further analysis has been required for some of the tables and figures.

DEMOGRAPHIC CHANGES

Since the beginning of the century, the population of England and Wales has grown from about 32.5 million to a little over 50 million. The increase was greatest in the first twenty years of the century — over 16 per cent. In the intervals 1921–41 and 1941–61 the population grew by about 10 per cent. The rate of growth slowed in the period 1961–81, and there was growth of only about 1 per cent in the period 1971–81. This growth in population was accompanied or partly triggered by a fall in mortality — the crude mortality rate declined during the century, and more particularly the overall mortality after adjustment for change in the age distribution of the population. Age-specific mortality trends throughout the century are shown in Figures 6.1 and 6.2; these indicate that there has been appreciable decline at

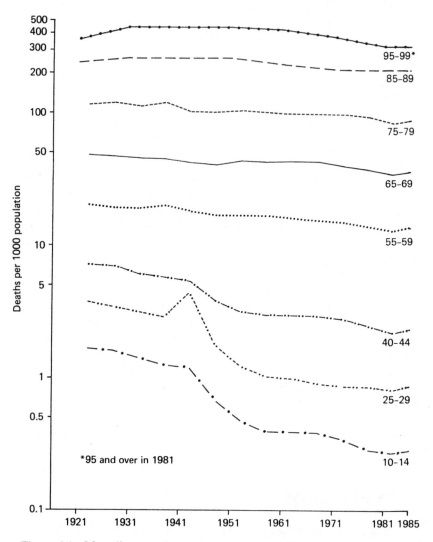

Figure 6.1 Mortality rates for males by age, England and Wales, 1921–85

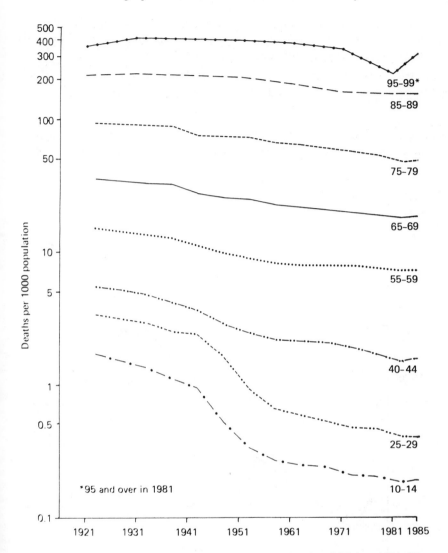

Figure 6.2 Mortality rates for females by age, England and Wales, 1921–85

younger ages, but less clear-cut decrease in mortality with advancing age in males (Office of Population Censuses and Surveys, 1985a). For females the initial mortality rates in the elderly were lower than in males, and they may have more clearly shown a decline throughout the century. With the decline in mortality, there has been an increase in the expectation of life; this has risen relatively steadily for both males and females, although the gain has been greatest for females, compared with males (Registrar General, 1914; Office of Population Censuses and Surveys, 1986). At the beginning of the century (1901–10) it was 48.5 years for males and 52.4 years for females, while the data for 1982–84 suggest that the expectation at birth is 71.6 years for males and 77.6 years for females.

MORTALITY

Figure 6.3 shows the age-specific mortality in males and females throughout the age range in 1985 (Office of Population Censuses and Surveys, 1987).

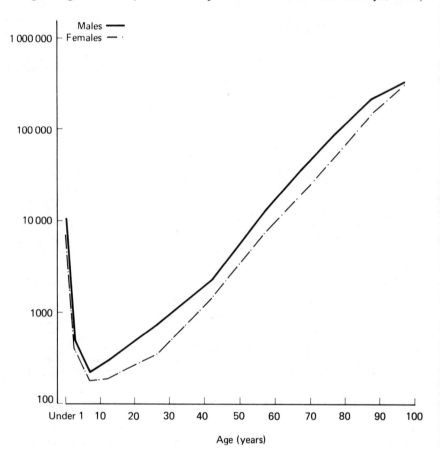

Figure 6.3   All-cause mortality rates per million population for males and females by age, England and Wales, 1985

There are high rates of mortality in the newborn, with relatively low rates existing up until early adult life. The rates then rise inexorably (the figure is plotted on a log scale and this steep rise with advancing age indicates a very marked increase in the force of mortality). Throughout the age-span of the elderly, the rates for males are higher than the rates for females (as already indicated in other material). Table 6.1 shows the five main causes of death in

Table 6.1 Main causes of death in males and females aged 60–84, England, 1984

Sex	Rank	Cause	%
Males	1	Ischaemic heart disease	33
	2	Lung cancer	11
	3	Cerebrovascular disease	10
	4	Digestive organs cancer	8
	5	Chronic obstructive pulmonary disease	8
Females	1	Ischaemic heart disease	27
	2	Cerebrovascular disease	16
	3	Digestive organs cancer	8
	4	Breast cancer	5
	5	Lung cancer	4

the age range 60–84 in males and females with the percentage that each of the causes represents of all deaths (Office of Population Censuses and Surveys, 1985b). The cause ranked first for both males and females is ischaemic heart disease — responsible for one-third of all deaths in males and a little over one-quarter of deaths in females. The second-ranked cause is lung cancer in males and cerebrovascular disease in females. This latter condition appears as the third cause in males, while malignancy of the digestive tract is the third cause in females. Again the latter condition is the next cause in males, while the fourth cause in females is breast cancer. The final cause for males is chronic obstructive pulmonary disease (including what was hitherto referred to as chronic bronchitis), with lung malignancy the fifth cause in females. These five causes account for 70 per cent of the deaths in males and 60 per cent of the deaths in females. If the table were extended, it would require many more causes to account for the next 20 per cent, as each succeeding cause accounts for only a very small proportion of the further deaths. It must be remembered that the causes can be grouped in various ways. Using 'all neoplasms' instead of specific sites of malignancy will radically alter the ranking in such a table.

Trends in mortality in the elderly have recently been examined, as part of an exercise in projecting future mortality (Alderson and Ashwood, 1985). The age-specific mortality rates from ischaemic heart disease have been disappointingly level throughout the period 1960–84 for both males and females. At ages 60–84 and over there has been virtually no indication of a decline in mortality. Rather different have been the trends for cerebrovascular disease, which for males and females shows a relatively steady decline in the mortality from 1950 onwards. There are parallel falls in the age-specific rates suggesting a period change in mortality, which some authorities have ascribed to control of hypertension (Acheson and Williams, 1983).

The cancers show a dismal picture; lung cancer is still rising for males in the oldest age group, although there has been a welcome cessation of the rise in the cohort born around the turn of the century (and alterations in the rates are anticipated, therefore, in the oldest age group in a few years' time). For females an increase is noted for all age groups in the elderly category — a reflection of the more recent spread of the smoking habit from males to females, and the fact that those now entering the elderly category have smoked more than the previous cohorts. For breast cancer, there is a very flat curve throughout the century in age-specific mortality, with no clear indication that early detection or treatment is having an impact upon this (although there may be an increase in incidence, partly due to changes in age at first pregnancy and other aspects of fertility, and improvement in survival balancing the increase in incidence). The main sites of malignancy in the gastrointestinal tract show some decrease during the century, particularly for stomach cancer. A worrying aspect of these trends is the cessation of the decline and more recent increase for oesophageal cancer.

Chronic respiratory disease in males aged 60–74 showed a welcome decline from the 1960s; the rates for females aged 60–84 showed a decline from the 1940s onwards, although this was less marked at the younger end of the age range, and now shows a rise in mortality (Alderson and Ashwood, 1985).

CANCER INCIDENCE

Since 1962 there has been a national scheme for registration of cancers which provides statistics of newly diagnosed malignancy at any age. These data are suitable for examining the age-specific incidence rates. These can be applied to a life table to indicate the probability of individuals developing malignancy with advancing age. The cumulative probabilities for all malignancies combined suggest that about one-third of males and females will develop some form of malignancy by the age of 90, and that about one-half of this incidence will have occurred by the age of 65.

The national system permits the calculation of the survival rates for individuals registered with different malignancies. These data can be examined by age at registration, and the survival can be corrected for the known life table survival in the different age groups. Despite this correction, there is appreciably lower survival in malignancy occurring in the very elderly compared with that in the middle-aged or the younger adult. The following comments deal with the sites of malignancy that have already been mentioned in the previous section. There is a low relative survival for lung cancer; this varies from 12 or 13 per cent in males and females aged 35–44, down to 5 or 7 per cent in those aged 85 and over (Cancer Research Campaign, 1982). Stomach cancer shows comparable survival. Colon cancer shows relative survival of one-third in younger adults but only 12 per cent for males or 19 per cent for females aged 85 and over. Very different is the relative survival in breast cancer, although again there is decreasing survival with advancing age; at ages 85 and over the relative survival is more than one-third at five years, while at ages 55–64 it is over one-half. (The relative survival is that observed after allowance for the deaths from all other causes.)

HOSPITAL IN-PATIENT STATISTICS

The Office of Population Censuses and Surveys process data for a 10 per cent sample of patients who have had in-patient care in NHS hospitals other than those for the mentally ill and mentally subnormal (for which the Department of Health and Social Security publish statistics). As with mortality, the statistics for hospital in-patient care show a marked rise with advancing age; this applies to the mentally ill and to other patients, excluding maternity (Alderson, 1983). This is so for the number of discharges, and also for statistics on occupied bed days (this is a statistic compounded of admission rates and length of stay, with the elderly having higher admission rates and also longer lengths of stay). Although the increase with advancing age is not so steep for hospital statistics as for mortality, it is linear on a log scale from the age of 30 onwards. Separation of the statistics by marital status shows lower rates for married females and males than for single and other categories of marital status.

Data on discharge diagnoses for in-patients (Department of Health and Social Security *et al.*, 1984) are used later on for comparisons with mortality and contact in primary care.

PRIMARY MEDICAL CARE

Three major studies have been carried out in collaboration with a sample of volunteer general practitioners and the support of DHSS, collecting information about GP contact with patients (Logan and Cushion, 1958; Royal College of General Practitioners *et al.*, 1974, 1986). The simplest statistic to examine is the contact rates, ignoring diagnosis. One way of highlighting the volume of care given to the elderly is to examine the percentage of all GP consultations that involve a home visit. This is higher in children under school-leaving age than in the main adult spans of 15–44 and 45–64. However, by age 65–74 nearly one-third of contacts with both male and female patients involve a home visit, while at age 75 and over nearly two-thirds of contacts with females are by way of a home visit.

Data are available on the diagnoses for which the patients are seen; the next section contrasts the pattern of contact in primary medical care with reasons for hospital admission, or causes of death. As will be readily understood, there are appreciable contacts for relatively transient disease not warranting hospitalisation. In addition, the family doctors shoulder a heavy burden of care in repeat contact with patients suffering chronic diseases — for whom they may care with or without support from hospital.

THE DIFFERENT PATTERNS OF DISEASE IN PRIMARY CARE, HOSPITAL IN-PATIENT CARE AND CAUSE OF DEATH

Table 6.2 sets out a comparison of mortality by cause, hospital discharge — that is, hospital discharge from hospitals excluding psychiatric and maternity — and diagnosis when consulting a general practitioner. (This uses the sources already discussed in the previous sections.) The table includes some of the conditions that have already been discussed and a number of other chronic diseases. For the age groups 65–74 and 75 and over, the percentage of all deaths, all hospital discharges and all consultations with a GP for these selected causes has been set out by sex. Comparison of the sets of figures indicates those conditions which are relatively common causes of death but cause fewer hospital discharges or GP consultations, and vice versa.

Thus, ischaemic heart disease is a very common cause of death in males and females in both the age groups examined, but accounts for an appreciably smaller percentage of discharges. The same applies to lung cancer; although the disparity between percentage of death and percentage of discharges is not so marked, there is an even lower figure for GP consultations. Some of the other conditions listed in the table show a higher percentage of discharges than deaths, while arthropathies and related disorders show much higher contact rates in primary medical care. The table is sufficient to indicate that the pattern of diseases associated with primary medical care and hospital care differs from the pattern of diseases causing death. This is partly due to the natural history or case fatality of the different diseases — some of which have relatively poor survival, while others, such as the arthropathies, are chronic disorders which are disabling but with low or very low mortality.

DISABILITY

An important issue in considering the health of the elderly is whether appreciable numbers of individuals living in private households are suffering

Table 6.2 Percentage of deaths in 1984, hospital discharges in 1982 and patients consulting GPs in 1981–82, for selected causes in males and females aged 65–74 and 75+, England

Cause	65–74 Males			65–74 Females			75+ Males			75+ Females		
	Death	discharges	GP	Death	discharges	GP	Death	discharges	GP	Death	discharges	GP
Lung cancer	12.1	4.2	0.9	6.1	1.5	0.2	6.8	2.5	0.9	1.7	0.5	0.1
Breast cancer	–	–	–	5.6	2.9	1.0	–	–	–	2.5	1.5	0.9
Hypertensive disease	0.8	0.4	16.6	1.0	0.6	20.2	0.7	0.2	10.3	0.9	0.4	12.9
Ischaemic heart disease	34.9	7.6	11.4	28.1	5.3	6.5	27.9	5.1	11.3	25.0	4.4	7.8
Cerebrovascular disease	9.3	4.7	2.1	12.8	4.5	1.7	12.7	6.2	5.1	18.7	7.1	4.2
Chronic obstructive pulmonary disease and allied conditions	7.1	3.7	12.0	4.1	2.4	5.5	8.5	4.1	12.4	2.5	1.5	4.2
Diseases of oesophagus, stomach and duodenum	0.8	2.0	3.0	0.9	1.9	2.0	1.0	2.1	2.7	1.1	1.9	1.7
Non-infective enteritis and colitis, and other diseases of intestines and peritoneum	0.6	1.8	5.2	1.1	3.1	6.2	0.8	2.1	7.2	1.4	3.1	7.7
Nephritis, nephrotic syndrome and nephrosis	0.5	0.5	0.5	0.6	0.4	0.3	1.1	0.7	0.5	1.1	0.5	0.5
Arthropathies and related disorders	0.3	2.1	11.6	0.8	4.9	20.6	0.3	1.7	13.1	0.9	4.1	23.1

from handicapping conditions. A major survey was carried out in Great Britain in 1968–69, which categorised the degree of disability of individuals reporting handicap. Data were presented by age, which showed that in the oldest age group of 75 and over, 7 per cent of males and 10 per cent of females report very severe handicap, with an additional 11 per cent of males and 15 per cent of females reporting severe handicap (Harris *et al.*, 1971). This indicates the prevalence of such conditions in people living in their own or their families' households. More limited data are collected now as a routine in the annual General Household Survey; this obtains respondents' views of any disability present (Office of Population Censuses and Surveys, 1985c). An appreciable proportion of individuals report limiting long-standing illness — the Survey in 1983 indicated that over two-thirds of males and females 75 and over considered that they had some form of limiting long-standing illness.

FACILITIES AND SUPPORT FOR THE ELDERLY

The census provides some indication of household amenities available, and it is possible to extract data for households that only include individuals over pensionable age. The material can be separated into those under and over 75, and this shows that an appreciably higher percentage of the very elderly are without a bath, or in households with outside toilets. For the country as a whole, less than 1 per cent of households do not have a bath, but this proportion rises to 3.8 per cent for those between pensionable age and 74, and to 6.1 per cent for those 75 and over. Only 1.6 per cent of all households have to use an outside WC, but this proportion rises to 4.8 per cent of those over pensionable age but under 75, and up to 7 per cent for those 75 and over.

The General Household Survey produces tables by age and sex on the percentage of individuals in private households using various facilities of personal social services. For example, 3 per cent of males and 6 per cent of females aged 65–74 had a home help visiting them in 1983, and this proportion rises to 28 per cent of males and 40 per cent of females aged 85 and over. Similarly, there are increases in the percentage having meals on wheels, but a rather different pattern in those attending a day centre. The highest proportion is 4 per cent of males and 8 per cent of females aged 75–84, with slightly lower figures both above and below this age range.

Table 6.3 represents an estimated distribution of the percentage of persons over pensionable age cared for by the health and welfare services on any given day in 1981. Using data from a variety of sources, this indicates the percentage who will see their family doctor, attend out-patients, be resident in local authority accommodation (Part III), be in-patients in general hospitals or in-patients in psychiatric hospitals (this table uses data from the

Table 6.3 Percentage of persons over pensionable age being cared for by health and welfare services on any given day in 1981

Age	Sex	GP	OP	Part III	General hospital	Psychiatric hospital	Total
65–74	Male	1.6	0.6	0.5	0.7	0.5	3.9
60–74	Female	1.8	0.6	0.5	0.7		4.1
75+	Male	1.9	0.6	3.1	1.7	0.9	8.2
75+	Female	2.0	0.5	5.8	2.0		11.2

sources noted in earlier sections plus DHSS, 1984). The data are presented by age and sex, and show an increase in contact with health and welfare services with advancing age, and a slightly higher contact rate for females than for males within each age band. Overall, it is estimated that just over 8 per cent of the male and 11 per cent of the female population aged 75 and over were having care from one of these facilities day by day during 1981. It must be remembered that estimates of contact with health and welfare services would be higher if the other services indicated in the previous paragraph (such as meals on wheels, home help and day centre contact) were included.

BEHAVIOUR

Although it would be useful to consider many facets of behaviour that directly influence health, readily available routine statistics only provide data on diet, alcohol consumption and smoking. The National Food Survey provides data on food expenditure by category of food and the age of the housewife (Ministry of Agriculture, Fisheries and Food, 1984). Although this does not clearly relate to the complete age-span of members within a household, it can be assumed that where the housewife is aged 65–74, or 75 and over, she is likely to be either living alone or living with her spouse, and less likely to be living with children and others. Abstracting data for key sources of nutrient indicates that there is a lower expenditure per person per week in the households where the housewife is 65–74 than in those where she is younger, and an even lower expenditure where the housewife is 75 and over. The total expenditure on food was £9.73 where the housewife was 55–64, £9.24 where the housewife was 65–74 and £8.34 where the housewife was 75 or over. This only provides tangential information from routine sources of decreased nutrient intake in the elderly; the lower expenditure is more marked for meat and cheese than for all other foods.

The General Household Survey provides limited data on reported alcohol consumption in households in relation to age and sex. The data are only available for those aged 65 and over as a broad age group, but this shows a lower percentage of moderate or heavy drinkers (moderate drinking is equated to consumption of 5 or 6 units of alcohol at least once a week, or more than 6 units once or twice a month, with even greater intake required for the heavier category). As would be expected with a lower proportion of moderate and heavy drinkers, there is a higher proportion of abstainers aged 65 and over — 11 per cent among males and 22 per cent among females, in contrast with 5 per cent for males and 12 per cent for females aged 45–64.

More detailed data are available on cigarette consumption, which have been published by age and sex for the earlier part of this century by the Tobacco Research Council (Lee, 1976) and for the past ten years or so from the General Household Survey (Office of Population Censuses and Surveys, 1985c). Combining these statistics shows that the male cohort born in 1905 had a lower tobacco consumption when aged 60–64 than the previous cohort, and this has continued as the birth cohort has aged. Succeeding male cohorts coming into the elderly age range born up until 1915 show steadily decreasing cumulative cigarette consumption. However, for females the age-specific data for those aged 60–64 or older show a steadily increasing trend in cigarette consumption up to the present time, and no cohort yet reaching the elderly age group has shown a peak in cigarette consumption. The importance of these differences between the sexes is that one would expect the more recent male cohorts reaching the age-span to have decreasing cigarette-associated disease, while in future years there will still be increase in smoking-associated disease occurring in elderly females. This may occur for the next forty years in women at ages 70–74 and over.

Statistics have been published on participation rates in a variety of leisure activities by age and sex, such as outdoor and indoor sports, outings, sightseeing, entertainment, cultural activities, home-based activities and hobbies. However, the relationship of such information to health is not so clearly a causal one but a reflection of health status.

POPULATION PROJECTIONS

Information on the size and age distribution of future populations is required in planning health, welfare and social security provision. There are many important issues of general and specific planning where such information is an important component, including life assurance and other financial aspects. In order to project the population estimates into the future, one requires as a starting point the age and sex distribution of the initial population. Then, as far as those living are concerned (that is, excluding initially the issues of projecting future births), one needs to estimate the future trends in mortality. As a start one can consider the past trends in mortality and the suitability of extrapolation of these past trends. By examining the trends for cohort or period trends, guidance can be obtained about the most appropriate way of extrapolation. However, past changes in mortality may not be a sound guide to future mortality. The two main aspects of future change are: (1) whether there will be appreciable alteration of the incidence of particular diseases due to alteration in population exposure to aetiological factors; (2) the very different possibility that there will be improvements in the survival rates for particular diseases. For example, over the past thirty years there have been dramatic changes in the incidence of infectious diseases in many countries and alteration in the case-fatality rate for those who develop the infections. It is not nearly so clear what the future holds for cancer or cardiovascular disease.

Alderson and Ashwood (1985) investigated the trends of mortality in England and Wales, as a base for considering projection of mortality for those aged 65 and over. The ten main causes of death having been considered, particular attention was directed to ischaemic heart disease, lung cancer and bronchitis/emphysema/asthma. For lung cancer, there was a close relation of cohort trends in mortality to past cumulative smoking, particularly for males. A model was fitted to these data, to project the future mortality, in relation to past and recent information on smoking habits by sex and age. However, there was no apparent relationship between past smoking and respiratory mortality in either sex. There was no evidence of cohort changes, and the trends were quite different for the two sexes. However, for air pollution data, measured in terms of smoke emissions, there was evidence of a relationship for males, but not so clearly of one for females.

Every two years the Office of Population Censuses and Surveys publish population projections for the constituent countries of the UK. Figure 6.4 shows the numbers of individuals aged 65–69 and over projected in the period 1983–2023 (Central Statistical Office, 1987). The upper age group is 90+, an open-ended group. The top curve shows an anticipated rise in the number of elderly over the next 15 years, then a slight decline, which lasts only 5–10 years and is then followed by a relatively steady increase in numbers of elderly up until 2023. It is particularly at the most advanced ages that the increase occurs, with all the accompanying burden of disease and requirement for support indicated in the preceding sections.

An earlier section commented on the relatively high proportion of the elderly that were female. The projections for the future suggest that the current preponderance of females may slightly fall over the coming forty years (Table 6.4). For example, in the oldest age group of 90 and over, there are at present about 25 males for every 100 females; by 2023 this proportion is projected to increase to about 35 males for every 100 females. This decrease in the female preponderance is due to the relative changes over time of the age-specific mortality rates for the two sexes throughout the age range.

Table 6.4 Projections of the elderly population, United Kingdom, 1983–2023 (1000s)

Age group	1983 Base	1984	1985	1986	1987	1988	1989	1993	1998	2003	2013	2023
Males												
65–69	1155	1099	1147	1195	1244	1297	1338	1217	1165	1152	1471	1405
70–74	1013	1015	1014	1000	969	916	873	1042	984	949	984	1170
75–79	662	677	688	695	701	706	709	644	746	711	701	931
80–84	323	337	350	360	370	381	391	414	382	455	438	482
85–89	110	114	120	127	135	143	150	174	194	183	224	241
90 and over	38	38	39	40	41	42	44	56	73	87	113	133
65 and over	3301	3280	3358	3417	3460	3485	3505	3547	3544	3537	3931	4362
Females												
65–69	1413	1342	1392	1445	1499	1557	1602	1425	1356	1324	1696	1618
70–74	1389	1389	1385	1363	1322	1252	1191	1389	1275	1219	1239	1470
75–79	1109	1124	1131	1134	1136	1138	1139	1030	1155	1066	1013	1324
80–84	717	736	751	764	776	789	802	819	747	852	771	812
85–89	341	352	368	382	393	407	419	457	483	446	494	498
90 and over	148	152	158	164	171	177	184	219	262	297	351	383
65 and over	5117	5095	5185	5252	5297	5320	5337	5339	5278	5204	5564	6105
All persons												
65–69	2568	2441	2540	2640	2743	2854	2940	2642	2521	2477	3167	3023
70–74	2402	2404	2399	2363	2291	2168	2064	2431	2259	2167	2223	2640
75–79	1772	1800	1818	1829	1837	1843	1848	1674	1901	1777	1714	2255
80–84	1040	1074	1101	1124	1147	1170	1192	1232	1129	1308	1209	1294
85–89	451	465	488	509	528	550	570	631	677	629	718	739
90 and over	186	190	197	204	212	219	227	276	335	385	464	517
65 and over	8418	8375	8543	8669	8757	8805	8842	8886	8822	8741	9495	10467

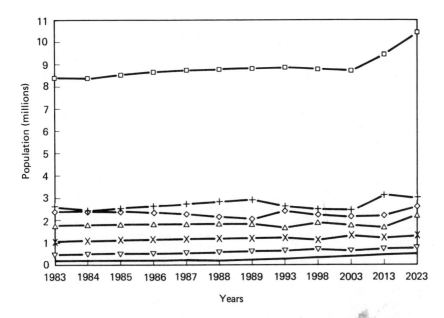

Figure 6.4 Population projections: persons aged 65–69 and above, UK, 1983–2023. □, Total; +, 65–69; ◇, 70–74; △, 75–79; ×, 80–84, ▽, 85–90; —, 90 and over

What is not evident from the basic projection is whether the improvement in mortality is associated with an increasing number of survivors who are healthy or with an increasing number of survivors who have chronic disease. It has already been shown that the patterns of diseases causing morbidity and mortality are very different; whether those with potentially fatal disease whose death is postponed have a higher prevalence of chronic disease is not revealed by the information at present available. This is a topic of importance upon which further work is required.

REFERENCES

Acheson, R. M. and Williams, D. D. R. (1983). Does consumption of fruit and vegetables protect against stroke? *Lancet*, **i**, 1911

Alderson, M. R. (1983). *An Introduction to Epidemiology*, 2nd edn. Macmillan, London

Alderson, M. R. and Ashwood, F. (1985). Projection of mortality rates for the elderly. *Pop. Trends*, **42**, 22

Cancer Research Campaign (1982). *Trends in Cancer Survival in Great Britain: Registrations 1960–74.* Cancer Research Campaign, London

Central Statistical Office (1987). *Annual Abstract of Statistics 1987.* HMSO, London

Department of Health and Social Security (1984). *The Facilities and Services of the Mental Illness and Mental Handicap Hospitals in England 1980–81.* HMSO, London

Department of Health and Social Security, Office of Population Censuses and Surveys, and Welsh Office (1984). *Hospital In-patient Enquiry*, main tables, 1982, England. Series MB4, No. 21. HMSO, London

Harris, A. I., Cox, E. and Smith, C. R. W. (1971). *Handicapped and Impaired in Great Britain.* HMSO, London

Lee, P. N. (1976). *Statistics of Smoking in the UK*, 7th edn. Tobacco Research Council, London

Logan, W. P. D. and Cushion, A. A. (1958). *Morbidity Statistics from General Practice*, Vol. 1: *General.* HMSO, London

Ministry of Agriculture, Fisheries and Food (1984). *Household Food Consumption and Expenditure: 1982* (Annual Report of the National Food Survey Committee). HMSO, London

Office of Population Censuses and Surveys (1985a). *Mortality Statistics: Serial Tables 1841–1980, England and Wales.* DHI, No. 15. HMSO, London

Office of Population Censuses and Surveys (1985b). *Mortality Statistics: Cause, England and Wales, 1984.* DH2, No. 11. HMSO, London

Office of Population Censuses and Surveys (1985c). *General Household Survey 1983.* HMSO, London

Office of Population Censuses and Surveys (1986). *Mortality Statistics, England and Wales, 1984.* DH1, No. 16. HMSO, London

Office of Population Censuses and Surveys (1987). *Mortality Statistics: Cause, England and Wales, 1985.* DH2, No. 12. HMSO, London

Registrar General (1914). *Supplement* to the *75th Annual Report of the Registrar General of Births, Deaths and Marriages in England and Wales, 1901–10.* HMSO, London

Royal College of General Practitioners, Office of Population Censuses and Surveys, and Department of Health and Social Security (1974). *Morbidity Statistics from General Practice 1970–71* (Second National Study). SMPS 26. HMSO, London

Royal College of General Practitioners, Office of Population Censuses and Surveys, and Department of Health and Social Security (1986). *Morbidity Statistics from General Practice* (Third National Study 1981–82). HMSO, London

Section 2
The Challenge of Providing for the Elderly

7

The Elderly as Members of Society: An Examination of Social Differences in an Elderly Population

Rex Taylor

INTRODUCTION

It is ironic that one of the unintended consequences of attempts to improve the circumstances and status of the elderly has been the tendency to describe them in an undifferentiated fashion. Ironic — but understandable: because the more those over a certain age are described as a group with shared experiences and deprivations, the more they are likely to obtain material improvements. While there can be no doubt that by comparison with younger age groups the elderly share a number of deprivations, this must not blind us to substantial differences between the elderly themselves. This chapter is concerned with the internal social differentiation of the distribution of personal resources — social, material, and mental and physical health — between age cohorts, sex groups and social classes. This is followed by a more focused examination of the distribution of these resources between a number of commonly identified risk groups — for example, those who live alone, the childless, recent movers. It ends with a more speculative examination of differentiation through the identification of lifestyle clusters.

AGE, SEX AND SOCIAL CLASS DIFFERENCES

Age

The distinction between the 'young' and the 'old' elderly is becoming increasingly important. Compared with those aged 65–74, those aged 75 and over have a greater number of long-standing health problems, they experience more illness and their use of services is twice, and in some instances four times, as great. We also know that the 'old' elderly are more likely to live in poorer housing and to have incomes below or on the margin of the State's standard of poverty. But in other respects we know that by comparison with their younger peers the 'old' elderly are advantaged: they have larger families, are more likely to have a child living in the neighbourhood and are generally more satisfied with their lives (Abrams, 1978, 1980).

Sex

The basis for many of the differences between elderly males and elderly females lies in differential life expectancy. At age 65 a Scottish woman can expect to live for another 15.7 years, whereas a Scottish man can only expect another 11.7 years (Registrar General (Scotland), 1982). As a result of this greater longevity, elderly women are twice as likely to be widowed and three times as likely to be living alone. Of course, elderly women are also more likely to live alone because they were less likely to marry in the first place, slightly more than 10 per cent of all women over the age of 65 being spinsters, whereas only 4 per cent of all men over the age of 65 are bachelors (Registrar General, 1978). These demographic differences between men and women have important financial consequences. In his discussion of poverty among the elderly, Townsend shows that those never married and those widowed have lower incomes and fewer assets than those currently married (Townsend, 1979). There are also consequences for social support, all men over the age of 65 being twice as likely as their female contemporaries to have a spouse and slightly more likely to have a surviving adult child (Shanas *et al.*, 1968). Health constitutes another source of inequality between the sexes. Elderly women report more long-standing health problems, they experience more illness and they report more GP consultations. Elderly women also seem to have poorer psychological functioning than do their male peers; they are more likely to suffer loneliness and anxiety, and to have weaker self-concepts and lower levels of morale/life satisfaction (Atchley, 1976).

Social Class

Compared with elderly from non-manual occupational backgrounds, those from manual backgrounds are less likely to have accumulated savings, property and private pension rights, and, as a consequence, they have lower net disposable incomes and lower net unit assets (Townsend, 1979). The best evidence for class differences in the health of the elderly comes from the General Household Survey (GHS). Taking the incidence of long-standing illness as the best single indicator of ill-health, recent reports show that, while the rates for those aged 65 and over show the same class pattern as is found in younger age groups, the gradient is less pronounced. Nevertheless, the overall evidence from GHS and other sources suggests that those from middle-class occupational backgrounds enjoy a clear health advantage in later life. Evidence for class differences in psychological functioning is rather sketchy. American researchers have consistently found a direct relationship between socioeconomic status and morale, but other dimensions have not received the same attention. The culture of poverty literature contains numerous studies suggesting working-class — particularly, lower working-class — disadvantage, but since most of these studies are descriptive, the evidence is, at best, suggestive and inferential. This catalogue of working-class disadvantage is partly offset by the working class's greater share of available family support. In the UK both Shanas *et al.* (1979) and Abrams (1978, 1980), in studies 20 years apart, have confirmed that, by comparison with their middle-class peers, working-class elderly have more children and more siblings, and are more likely to live with or near their close kin.

Age/Sex/Class Subgroups

While much is already known about the distribution of resources by age, sex and class, few researchers have considered the effect of these variables simultaneously. The combination gives rise to eight age/sex/class subgroups: 'young' middle-class males; 'young' middle-class females; 'young' working-class males; 'young' working-class females; 'old' middle-class males; 'old' middle-class females; 'old' working-class males; and 'old' working-class females. A range of detailed information is available in an earlier publication (Taylor and Ford, 1983b), and for present purposes it is sufficient to examine overall differences.

Table 7.1 is based on a random sample of the non-institutionalised elderly in Aberdeen and shows subgroup deviations from the sample mean for a range of resource variables. It is immediately apparent that only one subgroup is consistently better off than the sample as a whole — the group of younger working-class men. Younger middle-class males also emerge as an advantaged group, only falling below the sample mean in the availability of social support. The two groups of older females provide a sharp contrast, neither group ranking better than the sample as a whole on more than two out of the twelve resource variables. If we want to discriminate between these two groups to identify the one which is more disadvantaged, we have to examine each resource area in turn. For income, it is obvious that it is the working-class group which is massively disadvantaged. For social support, it is equally obvious that it is their middle-class peers who are most disadvantaged. As far as health is concerned, there is little difference between the two groups. For the final resource area — psychological functioning — the middle-class group has a slight overall advantage. The limitations of this

The Ageing Population

Table 7.1 Subgroup deviations from sample means (+ = better than; − = worse than)

	60–74				75+			
	Male	*Female*	*Male*	*Female*	*Male*	*Female*	*Male*	*Female*
Resource variables	M	M	W	W	M	M	W	W
Income	+16.61	+7.18	+2.41	−5.45	+2.78	−0.41	−5.44	−12.61
Currently married	+0.30	−0.10	+0.29	−0.01	+0.23	−0.35	+0.06	−0.35
Local children	−0.54	−0.39	+0.11	+0.45	−0.14	−0.63	+0.23	+0.22
Local siblings	−0.32	−0.27	+0.31	+0.39	−0.27	−0.48	−0.37	−0.33
Close friends	−0.07	+0.32	+0.32	−0.09	−0.01	+0.60	−0.45	+0.23
Chronic conditions	+0.74	+0.54	+0.48	−0.30	+0.36	−1.07	+0.15	−0.87
Symptoms	+0.70	+0.71	+0.56	−0.51	+1.07	−0.94	+0.19	−0.94
Functioning	+1.35	+0.93	+0.97	+0.52	+0.35	−2.89	−0.83	−2.17
Self-esteem	+0.73	+0.18	+0.39	−0.15	+0.92	−0.95	+0.06	−0.45
Self-competence	+1.62	−0.07	+0.19	+0.09	+0.31	−0.38	−0.15	−0.56
Morale	+0.23	−0.80	+1.02	−0.83	+2.54	+0.43	+0.89	−1.07
Health optimism	+0.76	+0.66	+0.06	−0.06	+0.20	−0.11	−0.90	−0.72

Notes: M = middle-class, W = working-class.

kind of approach notwithstanding, we therefore have to conclude that the older working-class females constitute the single most disadvantaged group.

RISK GROUPS

A more focused approach to differences within the elderly population can be obtained from an analysis of a number of commonly identified risk groups. The risk profile which will be presented for each risk group has its origins in the concept of 'personal resources' — i.e. those resources which individuals draw upon when coping with difficulties.

For present purposes nineteen key variables have been selected and arranged into six 'domains'. They have all been standardised to have a mean of zero and a standard deviation of unity. The score for the group on each variable is represented as a bar on a bar graph: a bar above the line represents a variable on which the average score for the group is above that of the sample as a whole, while a bar under the line represents a below-average score. The bigger the bar, the more different the group from the sample as a whole. Those scores on which the departure of the group from the sample mean is statistically significant are represented in the figures by stippling (Taylor and Ford, 1983a).

Those Living Alone

Accounting for about one-third of the elderly population, those living alone constitute the largest of the ten risk groups considered here. In our sample of 619 persons, 216, or 35 per cent, lived alone. They are disproportionately old, 40.5 per cent being aged 75 and over (as opposed to 29.7 per cent in the sample as a whole) and disproportionately female (80.3 per cent, as opposed to 60.7 per cent in the sample as a whole).

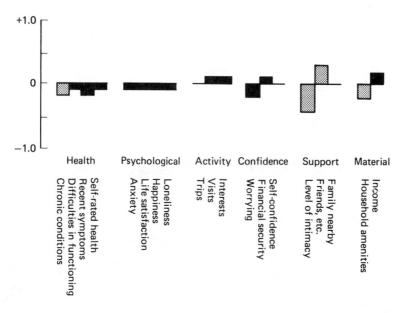

Figure 7.1   Living alone

For most of the measures of physical health, psychological functioning and confidence, it can be seen that, while the group scores slightly worse than the population as a whole, the only departure which is statistically significant occurs in the number of chronic conditions experienced. It is in relation to various forms of social support that those living alone differ most. They have fewer intimates or confidantes available to them, and, viewing their profile as a whole, this is the most distinctive feature. However, despite having few confidantes, the group is not characterised by low levels of psychological functioning. One reason for this may be the compensatory effect of many friends, those living alone having significantly more friends than the rest of the population. The only other significant departure from the sample mean occurs in relation to household amenities, those living alone being less likely to have such household amenities as hot water, fitted bath, etc.

Considering their profile as a whole, it can only be concluded that those living alone do not stand out as being significantly disadvantaged. Of course, it is a large and heterogeneous group, and encompassed within it are members of other risk groups — the single, the divorced/separated and the recently widowed — whose profiles will be examined later.

The Childless

Those without children constitute the second-largest of the ten risk groups. In the sample of 619 persons, 20 per cent (123) were childless. Compared with the rest of the elderly population, they are indistinguishable in terms of age and sex, but they are disproportionately middle-class — 55 per cent, as opposed to 35 per cent in the sample as a whole.

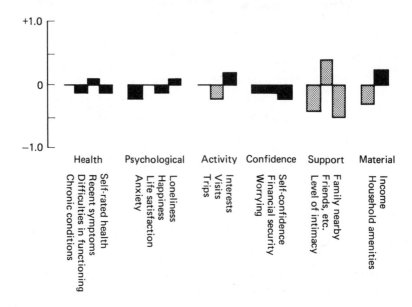

Figure 7.2   Childless

The most distinctive feature of their profile is found in the domain of social support. They have fewer intimates or confidantes and fewer family members living nearby, but this loss is partly compensated by the comparatively large number of friends. But being childless is not associated with levels of health, psychological functioning and confidence which are significantly lower than those pertaining in the elderly population. It is possible that they are slightly more anxious and have rather less self-confidence, but they just fail to achieve statistical significance on both measures. As far as social activities are concerned, they are significantly less likely to receive visits, and this is probably a direct consequence of being childless.

The reason for their comparatively poor showing on household amenities is not immediately apparent. However, children constitute a major incentive for such home improvements as installing a bath or an inside toilet, and they also provide local authority tenants with housing points in any attempt they might make to secure better accommodation. Thus, in a city such as Aberdeen, in which over 60 per cent of the housing stock is owned by the local authority, over the years the childless seem to have been left behind in the poorer inner-city areas, and they have to live with the consequences in their old age.

The Poor

Defining as poor those whose weekly income was below the Supplementary Benefit level identified a subgroup of 93, or 15 per cent of the sample. They are indistinguishable from the rest of the elderly population in terms of age and sex, but they are disproportionately from working-class backgrounds — 73.6 per cent, as opposed to 65.0 per cent in the sample as a whole. Widows are also overrepresented — 45.1 per cent, as opposed to 32.6 per cent in the sample as a whole. The married are underrepresented — 37.3 per cent, as opposed to 52.2 per cent in the sample as a whole.

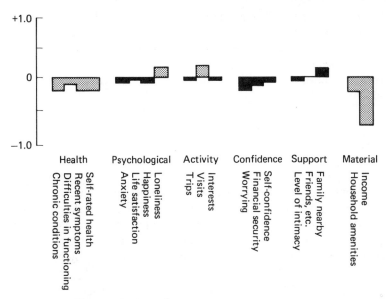

Figure 7.3 Poor (below Supplementary Benefit)

By comparison with the elderly population as a whole, they are clearly and massively deprived as far as income is concerned, but since this is the measure on which they are defined, the observation is completely tautologous. On the related measure, household amenities, they are also significantly worse off than the sample as a whole, but this could also be seen as rather tautologous.

Apart from being financially disadvantaged, the group is also rather comprehensively disadvantaged on health grounds, scoring significantly lower than the sample on all four health measures. This is an important finding, and additional analysis (not shown here) shows that the extent of health disadvantage is even greater among the poor who are widowed and divorced/separated. Turning attention to their mental health, evidence of risk or disadvantage is less conclusive. The group scores worse than the sample as a whole on all confidence measures, but the differences are not statistically significant; a similar situation pertains in respect of scores on anxiety, life satisfaction and happiness. The major exception — and this is statistically significant — occurs on the measure of loneliness. As a group, the poor are not as lonely as the rest of the elderly sample, and this finding is consistent with the rest of their profile. They receive significantly more visits than the sample as a whole, and they tend to have more family members living locally. These departures above the sample mean are clearly related: the poor are less likely to experience loneliness because they get more visits, and they probably get more visits because they tend to have more family members living locally.

On the basis of the data available, it is clear that the poor are not just disadvantaged in terms of their income and housing. Compared with the rest of the elderly population, they experience more illness and difficulties in functioning and have lower self-estimates of their health. However, it is important to note that this disadvantage is partially offset by their greater social contacts.

The Very Old

Almost 15 per cent of the sample (86 cases) were aged 80 and over. The group's composition is rather predictable, disproportionately female (74.1 per cent, as opposed to 60.7 per cent in the sample as a whole) and less likely to be currently married (19.5 per cent, as opposed to 52.2 per cent in the sample as a whole). They are also disproportionately from middle-class occupational backgrounds (40.4 per cent, as opposed to 35.0 per cent in the sample as a whole), but this result could have occurred by chance.

The risk profile of the very old generally confirms what is already known about their health; they have a greater number of chronic conditions and difficulties in functioning, and they tend to report more symptoms and to have lower self-ratings of their overall health. As a consequence, they make fewer daily trips outside the house, but they do not seem to have fewer visits made to them.

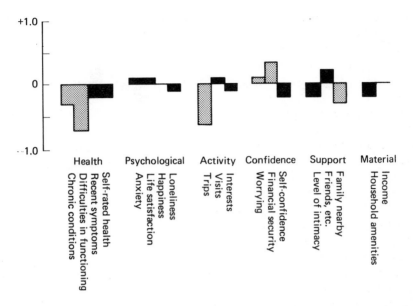

Figure 7.4   Very old (80 years and over)

On most measures of psychological functioning, the very old are either indistinguishable from the rest of the elderly population or are significantly better-off. It is clear that they worry less and feel greater financial security. This latter finding is of particular interest in view of the objective evidence that over half of the very elderly (80 years and over) have incomes below or on the margin of the State's standard of poverty. A number of factors might account for this discrepancy: for example, the very old may have fewer needs; income may have a lower salience for them than, say, health; or it may be that, by their own time perspective, present levels of provision seem generous.

The only other respect in which the very old are indisputably disadvantaged in relation to the rest of the elderly is the number of family members living locally. This difference is almost entirely explained in terms of differential survival. The very old are, by definition, survivors. Many of their siblings, and in some cases even their adult children, are not.

The Recently Moved

Contained within the sample were 85 elderly (13.7 per cent) who had moved home within the last two years. They are indistinguishable in terms of age, sex and marital status, but they are disproportionately from working-class occupational backgrounds (75.8 per cent, as opposed to 65.0 per cent in the sample as a whole). It is immediately apparent that most deviations from the

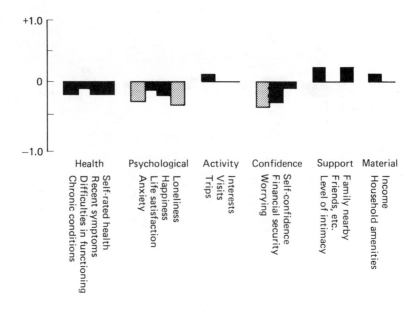

Figure 7.5   Recently moved

sample mean occur below the line, so that, as a group, they tend to be rather comprehensively disadvantaged. This disadvantage is particularly noticeable, and statistically significant, on three measures — anxiety, loneliness and worries — and containment within the psychological domain indicates the specific nature of the risks associated with residential mobility. It is worth observing that this psychological distress coincides with higher than average levels of intimacy and availability of family members.

The Recently Discharged

The sample contained 83 cases (13 per cent) who had been discharged from hospital in the two years preceding the interview. As a group, they are indistinguishable from the rest of the population in terms of age, sex, marital status and social class.

To define them as a risk group is partially tautological. They must all have been ill to enter hospital, and while some may have completely recovered after discharge, there will be many whose recovery is delayed, and some who never recover. But the frequency with which they are defined as a group at risk may also stem from more pragmatic considerations. Their entrances and exits from the hospital are documented, they are clearly identifiable, and they can (at least in theory) be routinely followed up as part of normal discharge procedure.

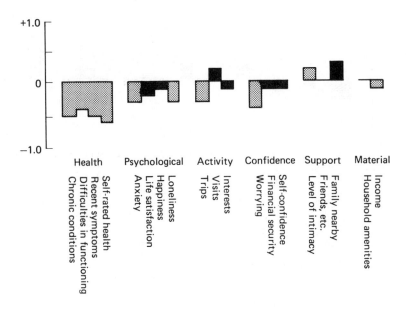

Figure 7.6   Recently discharged

Their profile is dominated by poor health. They score significantly worse than the rest of the sample on all measures of physical health and also on our psychological measures of anxiety, loneliness and general worrying. They also make significantly fewer trips outside the house, and have lower incomes. On the credit side, they report more confidantes and they tend to receive more visits and to have more family members living nearby. This is, therefore, a sense in which their physical and psychological condition mobilises higher levels of personal support than are available to the rest of the population.

Of all the risk groups so far examined, the recently discharged are clearly the most disadvantaged, and the profile merely underscores the need for follow-up services and support of various kinds.

The Never-married

The sample contained 70 cases (11.3 per cent) who had never married — 46 spinsters and 24 bachelors. Apart from containing a greater proportion of females (76.0 per cent, as opposed to 60.7 per cent in the sample as a whole), the group is also disproportionately middle-class (49.0 per cent, as opposed to 35.0 per cent). The most pronounced feature of their profile is found in the support domain. Compared with the rest of the elderly population, they have fewer confidantes and few family members living

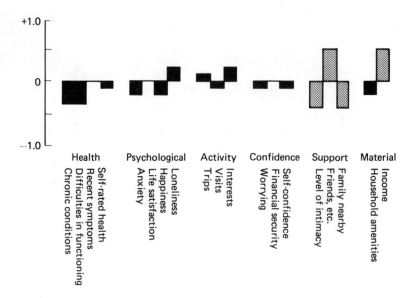

Figure 7.7   Never married

nearby. But, as already observed for other groups, there is clear evidence of compensation through friendship.

The Recently Widowed

The sample contained 202 widows and widowers, the majority of whom had been without their spouses for many years. Studies of widowhood have suggested that its psychological impact begins to tail off after about two years. Accordingly, 37 cases bereaved in the last two years have been identified as a potential risk group. Their profile reveals little conclusive evidence of comprehensive decline. Indeed, the only respect in which the group departs significantly from the sample mean is in their income, and here it can be observed that the departure is in a favourable direction. While departures on other measures fail to reach statistical significance, they come closest on happiness, trips out and worrying — all in the expected direction. But there are compensating tendencies, particularly in the confidence domain.

On the basis of the available evidence, this group cannot be claimed to be significantly disadvantaged by comparison with the rest of the elderly population.

The Isolated

While 216 of the sample members lived alone and, by definition, had no current spouse, 54 were additionally disadvantaged in having no children or

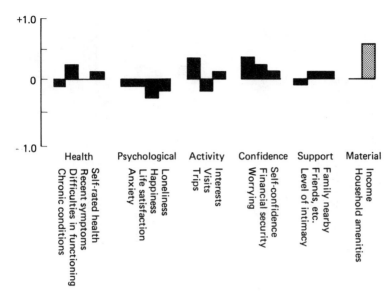

Figure 7.8 Recently widowed

siblings living locally. They have been defined as socially isolated. This group contains a higher proportion of the older cohort than the sample as a whole (48.1 per cent, as opposed to 29.7 per cent). It also contains more females (78.1 per cent, as opposed to 60.7 per cent), and more of those from middle-class occupational backgrounds (45.9 per cent, as opposed to 35.0 per cent).

It is clear from the group's profile that the disadvantage is fairly contained. With one exception, all significant departures from the sample mean occur in the support and material domains. Thus, apart from having poorer housing and better income, the isolated are not significantly different from the rest of the elderly population in any respect other than those by which they have been defined.

Social Class V

The sample contained 51 men and women (8.2 per cent) whose previous occupations qualified them for membership of the Registrar General's Social Class V. On other structural variables — age, sex and marital status — this group is indistinguishable from the sample as a whole.

It is clear from the group profile that Social Class V members are only significantly disadvantaged in terms of income. On all other measures, apart from one, the group cleaves fairly closely to the sample mean. The exception is the number of family members living nearby. Whatever disadvantage members of Social Class V may experience in health or psychological

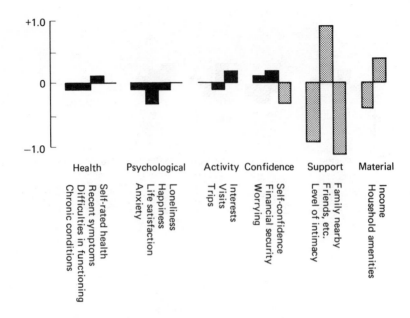

Figure 7.9 Isolated (no spouse or near family)

functioning, and there is not conclusive evidence in the data, the family support available to them is significantly greater than that enjoyed by the rest of the elderly population.

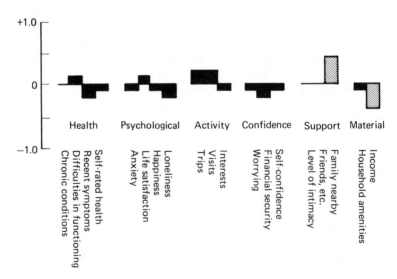

Figure 7.10 Social Class V

Summary

For summary purposes, it is convenient to identify three categories of risk group. Those minimally disadvantaged comprise the isolated, the never-married and, to a lesser extent, the childless. Compared with the rest of the sample, they all have little social support available to them, however, and this is the most important point; their disadvantage in the domain of social support does not 'spill over' into other domains. There is no evidence that their health or psychological functioning is worse than that of the sample as a whole. It is also important to note the way in which friends compensate for confidantes and family nearby.

The recently widowed, those living alone, the poor and those from Social Class V constitute a second category. They cleave rather closely to the sample mean, and are characterised by deviation both above and below. In resource terms, they have both strengths and weaknesses, an ambivalence rather clearly indicated in the resource profile of those defined as 'poor'.

The final category, consisting of the recently moved, the recently discharged and the very old, is characterised by those with more deviations below than above the sample mean. Moreover, and most important, they all score worse than the sample as a whole in terms of health and/or psychological functioning. These are clearly the groups at greatest risk.

LIFESTYLE CLUSTERS

Both of the approaches summarised above have proceeded on the basis of predefined groups. An alternative, and more exploratory, approach is possible through cluster analysis, which divides a sample into subgroups according to their similarity across a range of variables (Ford and Taylor, 1984). It is an entirely empirical and a theoretical procedure, but it does have the capacity to identify totally unexpected lifestyle patterns and groupings. The ten clusters identified are displayed according to the conventions outlined earlier (p. 108).

It can be seen at a glance that the first cluster consists of a highly favoured group, since all but two of the scores are above the mean. All scores above the mean are statistically significant. It constitutes an *elderly élite*. Reference to the structural data (not shown above) reveals that this first cluster is disproportionately male, from the younger cohort, married and middle-class.

The pattern of resources in Cluster 7.2 is very different and the whole profile is dominated by a single variable — availability of family living nearby. On most of the other variables, this cluster scores relatively close to the mean, except that they have significantly fewer difficulties in functioning and that they are also rather active outside the home. They are low on

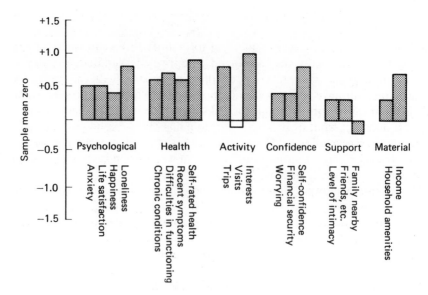

Cluster 7.1   'Elderly élite' (*n* = 107)

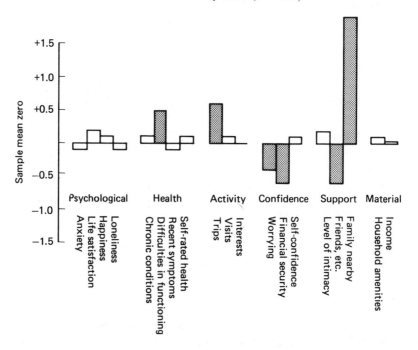

Cluster 7.2   'Family shielded' (*n* = 63)

friends, and this inverse relationship between family and friends seems to indicate a substitutive principle, since it is repeated in many of the clusters. They are also low on the worrying and security variables. The relevance of this pattern of resources is evident: they have high social support on which to draw in facing future hazards — i.e. *family shielded*. Unlike those in Cluster 7.1, they do not rank high on many of the other resource variables. Of all the clusters, this is the most homogeneous from a structural point of view; they are virtually all in the youngest age group and a considerable majority have a spouse. From a developmental perspective, Clusters 7.1 and 7.2 are both at the start of the passage through the vicissitudes of old age, but they each carry with them different patterns of handicap and resources.

Cluster 7.3 is another cluster where a very high score on one variable is the key to the cluster identity. In this case it is the visits variable which takes on an extreme appearance. Members are highly sociable within their own

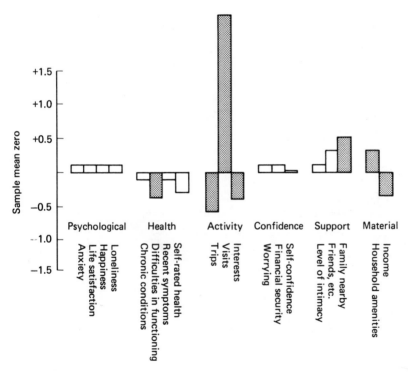

Cluster 7.3 'The supported' ($n = 33$)

homes. By contrast, they score low on trips out of the home and on physical functioning (as measured by number of difficulties in functioning). Not surprisingly, in view of the high interaction levels, they have above-average family support, but in other respects they are unremarkable. Structurally, they tend to be older than the sample as a whole, with a high proportion living alone. This is a group with a degree of impairment, but they are coping well by mobilising networks of sociability. Accordingly, it is appropriate to call them *the supported*.

Cluster 7.4 represents the first of the groups which is ageing unsuccessfully. They score below average on a large proportion of measures, particularly those dealing with health, psychological well-being and activities. Again, like Cluster 7.3, a large number of functioning difficulties seems to go with restricted activity outside the home, but in this case the degree of impaired functioning is greater, and there is no compensatory socialising within the home. Cluster 7.4 has a high proportion of females and widows, with the most numerous group being old, middle-class widows. Accordingly, they are referred to as the *ill and unsupported*.

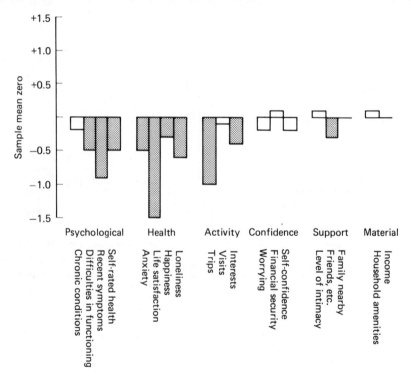

Cluster 7.4   'Ill and unsupported' (*n* = 50)

Cluster 7.5 is, at first glance, rather impenetrable, with no very extreme scores and a selection above and below the mean. On closer inspection, one can see a pattern of high intimacy through marriage, associated with rather low activity levels and social support (other than from the spouse). Scores on

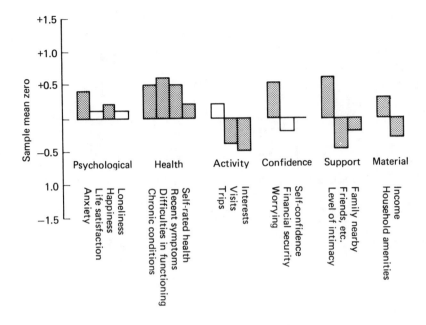

Cluster 7.5 'Exclusive couplehood' (*n* = 94)

other variables are generally favourable. Structurally, this cluster has a high proportion of males, the highest proportion married of any cluster (80 per cent) and a very low proportion living alone (13 per cent). This pattern might be described as successful ageing through *exclusive couplehood*.

Cluster 7.6 shows an interesting pattern. Here is a cluster in which health and psychological functioning are inversely related. Despite rather poor health, this group appears to have achieved high morale. Looking at the remaining variables, it can be seen that they have many friends and a high level of interests and hobbies, but a low level of family support. They also worry rather a lot. Structurally, they are female and disproportionately old. This is a group of *health optimists*. This inverse relation of health and psychological well-being is of considerable interest. They appear to have successfully mobilised interests and friendships to compensate for problematic health.

Cluster 7.7 contrasts dramatically with Cluster 7.6 and is a group with poor psychological health, which is probably not explained by the remaining variables. The health variables are not generally low, with the exception of recent symptoms, and this might well be due to the inclusion of certain psychosomatic symptoms in the symptom list. Activities are mixed, with trips above average and visits below. They are rather low on family and friends. Not surprisingly, they are also low on 'confidence' variables. They

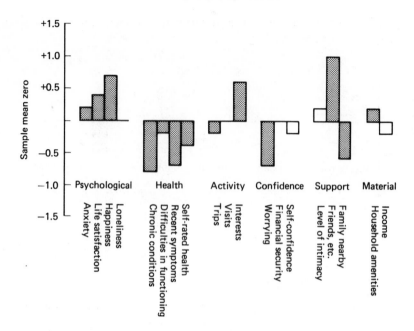

Cluster 7.6 'Health optimists' (*n* = 73)

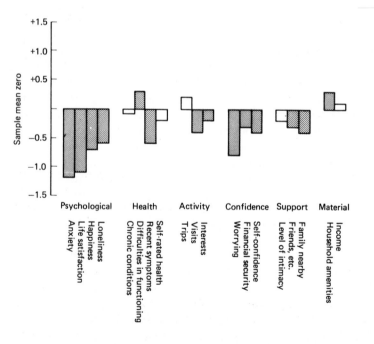

Cluster 7.7 'Psychologically fragile' (*n* = 67)

worry, feel insecure and have low confidence in their own potency. They can be called the *psychologically fragile*.

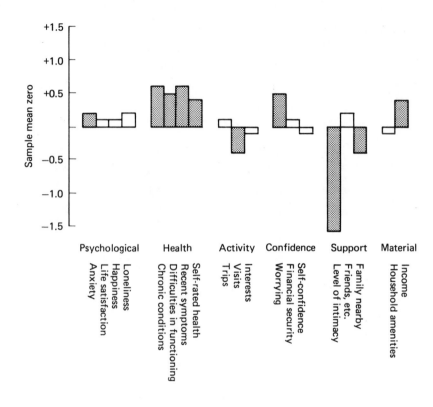

Cluster 7.8 'Socially isolated but defended' (*n* = 67)

Cluster 7.8 is, again, characterised by one very distinctive variable. This group scores very badly on intimacy. They have no one with whom they feel they can share their feelings. As we might expect, they have few family nearby. They receive few visitors, but, apart from this, they score well. They have average psychological well-being, and above-average health. They do not worry, and they enjoy above-average income. Provisionally, they can be described as *socially isolated but defended*.

Cluster 7.9 has the most unusual profile of all our clusters and is defined almost exclusively in terms of poor housing conditions. It is a group of inner-city tenement dwellers living in totally inadequate housing. (Their scores were so low that we checked the original schedules.) They also have low incomes and few interests, but, despite these handicaps, they seem

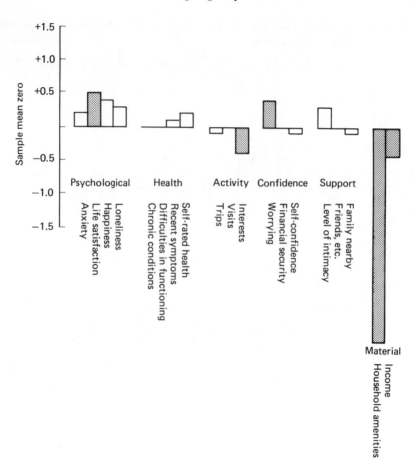

Cluster 7.9 'Inadequately housed' (*n* = 25)

highly satisfied with their lives and they are significantly less likely to worry than other sample members. Structurally, they are older than the rest of the sample, and a high proportion live alone. The most obvious name for the cluster is the *inadequately housed*, but this is not very revealing.

Cluster 7.10 is the mirror image of Cluster 7.1. They are in jeopardy in almost every way. They have extremely poor health, poor psychological functioning and low confidence. They do have slightly above-average family support, and it seems that this might be reflected in the number of visits they receive. Their health and psychological scores are very low. They are markedly female, old and working-class, and a considerable proportion live alone. In the Scottish vernacular, they would be called *poor souls*.

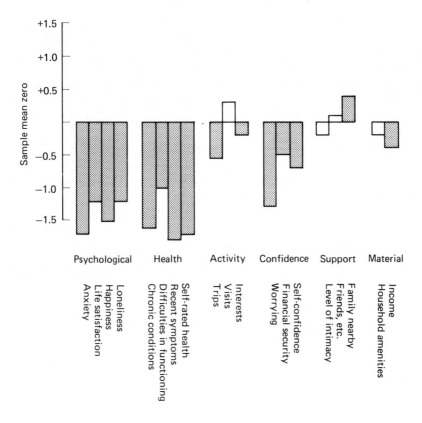

Cluster 7.10 'Poor souls' ($n = 39$)

CONCLUSION

Throughout this chapter the aim has been to illustrate ways in which the elderly population is differentiated. It started with an exploration of structural differentiation, showing how personal resources vary by age, sex and social class. This was followed by a more focused examination of the distribution of personal resources in a number of risk groups, some structurally defined (e.g. the single, recent movers). The voluntaristic component was stronger in the third section, where the patterning of personal resources was examined, to reveal a number of distinct lifestyles.

In the introduction to this book the editors have adopted what they call a 'positive' orientation towards ageing and the elderly. The orientation of this chapter has been neither positive nor negative, but, it is hoped, realistic. Whatever the elderly have in common, they are different from each other in much the same ways as any other age group. Moreover, many of the differences existing in old age are the outcome of earlier differences. Put another way, the personal resources available to meet the vicissitudes of old age do not come with a pension book. They are rooted in earlier choices and constraints in employment; number and spacing of children; composition and strength of the peer group; hobbies and interests; and so on. These realities have long been accepted by psychologists, and the present chapter should be read as a sociological analogue of a psychological exploration of individual differences.

Finally, while much of the work reported in this chapter is fairly exploratory and requires confirmation from other studies, it will be apparent that it could have important implications for practice and policy. For practitioners, the highly differentiated pattern of personal resources and lifestyles could provide clues to a better understanding of responses to such role transitions as widowhood, retirement and disability. For practitioners and policy-makers, there are also implications at the level of resource allocation. In conditions of scarcity of most resources — domiciliary visits, home helps, special housing, institutional places — allocation decisions have to be guided by a differential gerontology. The more that is known about the ways in which the elderly differ, the greater the possibilities of targeting resources to those in greatest need.

ACKNOWLEDGEMENT

The research reported in this chapter was done jointly with Graeme Ford of the MRC Medical Sociology Unit, Glasgow.

REFERENCES

Abrams, M. (1978, 1980). *Beyond Three Score Years and Ten* (First and Second Reports on a Survey of the Elderly). Age Concern England, Mitcham
Atchley, R. C. (1976). Selected social and psychological differences between men and women in later life. *J. Gerontol.*, **31** (2), 204
Ford, G. and Taylor, R. C. (1984). Differential ageing: an exploratory approach using cluster analysis. *Int. J. Ageing Hum. Dev.*, **18** (2), 141
Registrar General (Scotland) (1982). *Annual Reports*. Edinburgh
Shanas, E., Townsend, P., Wedderburn, D., Friis, H., Stenhouwer, J. and Milhø, J. P. (1968). *Old People in Three Industrial Societies*. Routledge and Kegan Paul, London
Shanas, E., Townsend, P., Wedderburn, D., Friis, H., Stenhouwer, J. and Milhø, J. P. (1979). *Old People in Three Industrial Societies*. Routledge and Kegan Paul, London, later edition
Taylor, R. C. and Ford, G. (1983a). The elderly at risk: a critical examination of commonly identified risk groups. *J. Roy. Coll. Gen. Pract.*, **33** (256), 699

Taylor, R. C. and Ford, G. (1983b). Inequalities in old age: an examination of age, sex and class differences in a sample of community elderly. *Ageing and Society*, **3** (2), 183

Townsend, P. (1979). *Poverty in the United Kingdom.* Penguin, London

8

The Role of the Charitable and Voluntary Organisations

David Hobman

INTRODUCTION

The term 'voluntary sector' embraces a wide range of non-statutory organisations involved in providing services for old people, in representing their interests and in making their views heard. It is sometimes wrongly confused with privatisation by both its critics and its supporters. It serves a different purpose, although in a pluralist society, with a mixed economy, it provides one of the elements through which personal choice can be made available to people who might otherwise be denied it. It also offers a means of participation and self-determination to both individuals and groups.

Although the voluntary sector's contribution is massive in terms of the human and financial resources it can command, nobody knows the precise size or extent of its contribution. It is difficult to qualify it and impossible to quantify it in crude terms of man-hours served, or public funds secured or saved, simply through the cataloguing of the alternative provisions it offers to those available through agencies of central or local government. This is because part of their cost still comes from the public purse in one form or another. For example, through tax or rate relief.

Whatever criteria are used to measure the extent of the voluntary movement's total contribution, it will be seen to represent a major force, although the individual elements which comprise it may sometimes operate in small isolated units without an apparent connection to any grand design or overall strategy. The National Council of Voluntary Organisations and its local constituents, the Councils of Voluntary Service and Rural Community Councils, play a useful role as intermediaries for those agencies wishing to co-operate, but their powers and influence over their constituents are limited. They can apply no sanctions to those who step out of line. In a similar way, Age Concern England (the National Old People's Welfare

Council) and its local constituents provide a catalyst for organisations working in their specialised fields.

The vibrancy and strength of the voluntary movement stems, in part, from its spontaneous eruptions of energy and its spirit of independence, as well as from the multiplicity of groups to be found within it. They range from those involving a considerable element of discipline, the wearing of a common uniform, to those which run free and are based on a substantial element of informality. But in spite of its idiosyncratic nature, and the great variety of its manifestations, there is a coherence about this central feature of the British way of life in the sense that it makes it possible for countless men and women from all social classes and of different ages to find an effective means of self-expression.

Another source of its energy and persistence in arguing for reforms, as well as actually providing alternative solutions as models of good practice, lies in the degree to which the majority of its most active supporters are committed to their causes. Better services for the housebound, increased allowances for carers, protection of those who are vulnerable, perhaps. But each cause is, in one sense, competing with others in the same field as well as with general ignorance, apathy or hostility. As a result, the voluntary sector is often highly competitive, and a co-ordinated approach is sometimes difficult to achieve. In the field of ageing, it is one of the primary functions of Age Concern, nationally and locally, to provide a catalyst for joint social action where bridges can be made between the sectors and where common causes can be identified and pursued.

THE SCOPE AND NATURE OF THE VOLUNTARY SECTOR

In order to understand the full scope of the voluntary sector, and its nature, it is first necessary to identify the major groupings which are to be found within it. At one end of the spectrum, they reflect traditional service-providing charities with an exclusive, or major, interest in old people. They operate on a national basis and their local constituents may be branches which follow central directions through a system of devolved management, or they may represent a network of autonomous self-governing local groups combining to form a federal organisation in which values are shared, but in which the nature of actual responses and priorities will differ in relation to local circumstances. In a secular sense, it could be described as the difference between the Established Church and non-conformity.

Voluntary societies which are based on central direction, through branch activities, are most likely to concentrate on service delivery and may include some case-work. In some cases, their roots may go back to the nineteenth century or even earlier. But even if their origins are more recent, they reflect the long tradition of philanthropic service in which those whose financial and personal circumstances are relatively secure and stable work among those who are disadvantaged. In this sense, they predate some of the agencies of the Welfare State. Indeed, many public health and social services have evolved from their pioneering activities. Religious organisations also represent a central part of this historic strand of British social life. Their existence constantly affirms the importance of the contribution which ordinary people can make to the educational, health and social services. Few government reports have failed to recognise their value. Their authors clearly understood that without their input many plans for social enhancement would be totally unrealistic.

In recent years, there has even been a shift among those with an idealistic commitment to a far greater degree of state or municipal involvement, although, where this is the case, grant-aid in support of voluntary action, or its right to exist, is likely to be associated with increased control over its activities. Some local authorities are now beginning to set out the strict terms on which voluntary service will be allowed to function in their areas of interest if it is to be in any way associated with public sector provisions.

Public acknowledgement of the central role of the voluntary sector in the general scheme of things during this century can be found in a whole series of reports ranging from Royal Commissions to Committees of Enquiry.

In 1909 all the members of the Poor Law Commission acknowledged that voluntary organisations were responsible for much valuable pioneering work. The signatories to the Minority Report went so far as to say that they thought 'it should be a cardinal principle of public administration that the utmost use should be made of voluntary organisations and the personal services of men and women of goodwill'.

Nearly fifty years later, after the birth of the Welfare State, another report on charitable trusts (Anon., 1952), which arose out of William Beveridge's book entitled *Voluntary Action* (Beveridge, 1948), expressed the same ideas when it said: ' . . . state action and voluntary action are not the antithesis of each other; rather they sprang from the same roots, were designed to meet the same needs and had the same motivating force behind them — indeed historically, state action is voluntary action crystallised and made universal'.

Again, more recently, the Seebohm Report on the Personal Social Services (Anon, 1968) repeated the same argument when it said: ' . . . the maximum participation of individuals and groups in the community in the planning, organisation and provision of social services is essential'. It also developed this theme of consumer participation, in which the users of the social services were seen as having a more active role than before. Although the Seebohm Report argued that the major recruitment of volunteers should be through voluntary organisations, it foresaw a considerable increase in their direct use by local authorities. It also made reference to the need for skills in developing this community resource to the full.

VOLUNTEERS — THEIR RECRUITMENT AND CONTRIBUTION

Indeed, the issue of volunteers became so important that a Committee of Enquiry was established by the (then) National Council of Social Service under the chairmanship of Dame Geraldine Aves, to explore the place of the volunteer in the social services. As a result of the report of that Committee (Anon., 1969), a new agency, The Volunteer Centre, was established in 1973 with the object of becoming a catalyst for all those who had an interest in the recruitment and development of volunteers in a wide range of settings. As the Seebohm Committee had anticipated, many of these volunteers were to be found working for public authorities, in a variety of roles, although the voluntary sector as a whole continues to be vigorous and to have developed very substantially in the last twenty-five years.

The growth of the movement of volunteer bureaux throughout the country providing the equivalent of job centres for uncommitted volunteers searching for something with which to occupy themselves which will meet their own interests and available time, is a testimony to the sense of partnership which has been evolving during the last twenty-five years, although the quality of the relationships between voluntary agencies and statutory authorities, as well as between them and organisations of professional or paid workers, varies widely from genuine understanding about their different, but complementary, roles to ambivalence or even distrust.

In this connection, some very valuable guidelines were prepared for The Volunteer Centre by a group of representatives of major voluntary organisations and trade union leaders, who set out the basis of sensible relations which could serve in normal times as well as in periods of industrial dispute when those at the receiving end of care services were most likely to be the victims. These guidelines included the following passages:

On the need to involve providers and consumers
Because local situations vary enormously, full consultation between management, staff organisations, representatives of volunteers and, where appropriate, through established channels for representatives of those receiving the service should take place. In this way decisions on the nature and extent of voluntary action can take account of the interests of all concerned and result in better all-round service.

On the need for clear understanding
The methods of communication can vary widely (written or spoken word) but well thought out agreements can founder if all the people associated with the representatives reaching the agreement are not clear on its nature, extent and practical application.

On the essential contribution of the volunteer
Voluntary work should not be used as a substitute for the work of paid staff, but

should instead complement it. The practical implications of this statement need to be discussed at local level. Whilst some tasks currently performed by volunteers would be performed by paid staff if resources were available, there are other activities, such as befriending, which in many cases can only be carried out fully by someone seen by the receiver of the service to be unpaid. We recognise, however, that paid staff are able to act from a mix of motives and offer friendship to clients even though they are being paid to be on duty. Likewise volunteers act from mixed motives. Volunteers should not threaten the work of paid employees, nor feel exploited as unpaid substitutes by the organisation where they are offering their service. Some volunteers may prefer to work to a clear job description, outlining clearly the work they may be required to undertake, with guidelines as to when this is appropriate.

On voluntary work and its impact on paid service
There have been occasions in the past where, without proper consultation, voluntary activity has been implemented which has threatened the jobs of paid staff and/or has had repercussions on earning levels. Such action, however well-meaning or intended, can only lead to a deterioration in the level of industrial relations and result in a poorer service. However, there will be situations in which organisational changes incorporating new notions of care might involve the use of volunteers in ways which could affect the interests of groups of paid employees. For example, new forms of voluntary care, such as the development of small group homes in the community for the mentally ill, thereby permitting the closure of wards in psychiatric hospitals, might remove the need for certain kinds of paid staff input. In this situation negotiations should take place with the relevant staff organisations with a view to reaching agreement to safeguard their interests. In this way new social policy initiatives, advantageous to the receiver of the service, can be implemented without any concomitant disadvantages to the staff.

On payment
Although volunteers should not normally receive financial reward, the group recognises that in a number of situations it is common practice to pay out-of-pocket expenses to volunteers.

On the value of a co-ordinator
It is an advantage to name an individual responsible for the co-ordination of voluntary work within an institution to whom paid staff can refer in the first instance if they feel that the guidelines are being overstepped; and to make clear that normal negotiating machinery is also available if necessary for settling problems in this field.

During industrial disputes
Any departure from normal work should only take place with the agreement of management and those staff organisations involved in the dispute.

Unfortunately, the tense situation between the Government and trade unions in the public sector during the winter of discontent (1978/79) brought further discussions of this important group to an end and more recent attempts to revive it have failed to re-establish a focus for an important dialogue.

In the mid-1960s a government publication (Hobman, 1965) began to catalogue services and the basis on which volunteers were recruited in very general terms. Now the process is infinitely more sophisticated. Employees of voluntary workers have had to spell out the conditions of service quite precisely in order to include minimum hours required, skills demanded, preparation and supervision given, and — of increasing importance to those with limited incomes — the basis on which travel or out-of-pocket expenses can be met.

The question of payment to volunteers remains a sensitive issue, and opinions are still sharply divided between the rapidly declining group who believe that any payment somehow invalidates the voluntary principle and the growing majority of people who understand that changing economic circumstances make it essential. This is particularly important when volunteers may themselves be retired people and in receipt of modest incomes which allow no margins for expenditure on anything but the essentials of daily living.

Indeed, with the rapid growth of widespread unemployment, government-funded programmes now recognise that voluntary service may offer a dignified, if temporary, opportunity for useful and, in some cases, learning experiences for people to undertake while out of work when they can apply existing skills or be helped to learn new ones. The major government programme, Opportunities for Volunteering, administered through a number of national networks, has played a useful part in the process since it has been acknowledged that those involved must expect reasonable financial returns and must be in a position to take permanent paid work in the normal way if, and when, opportunities present themselves.

Although this combination of volunteers, who reflect the more traditional approach and require no financial return, and those who may need a modest payment is thought to be a product of contemporary society, there are already a number of interesting precedents — for example, in the field of child-fostering, where families have been paid relatively small sums to make it possible for them to perform this valuable service on behalf of the community. In the same way, the development of good-neighbour schemes involving people in providing sustained support through regular visits to frail elderly neighbours living alone throughout the day and, in some cases, at night as well, or in providing an additional place at midday meal-tables, must involve at least acknowledgement of the costs incurred with reasonable margins. Indeed, it may well be within this field of sustained good-neighbourly care that a form of service to the community by its own members is going to be most crucial and effective in the coming years, given the number of very frail people living alone in their own homes into extreme old age. Social mobility and the early separation of generations have deprived many elderly people of a critical service which could be described in terms of tending to their personal needs. This is neither nursing nor domestic service, provided through the home help system, but it may be central to the new support networks designed to replace those once associated with the extended family.

THE RANGE OF VOLUNTARY SERVICES

So the picture builds up of people giving service to others on a formal basis, through organisations designed for the purpose to informal acts of good-neighbourliness which reflect a form of voluntary service, but which may be orchestrated through a statutory agency. It clearly takes many forms and calls upon the application of every type of knowledge. The housewife with her specialised experience of home management has just as much to offer as those with other skills and specialised training. In this context, it is mainly concerned with long-standing relationships by home visitors, car drivers, club organisers, or it may be concerned with short-term encounters. For example, through the provision of welfare rights information, or staffing of advisory centres; through counselling in relation to specific problems — for instance, bereavement. In these more specialised operations, the volunteers will be carefully selected, prepared and supervised for sensitive tasks which require identifiable knowledge and skills.

The value of personal service given through voluntary agencies, or by volunteers, does not lie simply in its scale of economy, which often has political attractions, but in the fact that support given within the community by its own members to those who live nearby is a practical expression of a commitment to the creation of a caring society. It is central to the implementation of any realistic and dynamic policy of community care. It is not a case that volunteers possess some quality not present in professional or paid workers, but because volunteers may be more regularly available and because in some instances help provided on this basis may be more acceptable, it may lack some of the stigmatisation associated with responses by the social services, for instance. Here the social worker or statutory officer may in some way be associated in the minds of older people with some of the indignities they can still remember from childhood of visits by the representatives of charities, wanting to separate the deserving poor from those who were assumed to have brought ruin or distress upon themselves through their own fecklessness. Much the same applied to the often crude administration of the official Poor Law services given on behalf of parishes by the representatives of the Guardians.

A circular issued by the (then) Ministry of Health (now Department of Health and Social Security), which the author of this chapter helped to compile, listing the tasks performed in the home and community nearly twenty-five years ago, would need few alterations to apply with equal force in a contemporary context. It included the relevant personal services provided to the individual at home and in the wider community shown in Tables 8.1 and 8.2.

Perhaps the only major difference now lies in greater specialisation on the part of some voluntary organisations: for example, in Crossroads schemes, work for the hard of hearing, heating and insulation, carers' support groups, teas-on-wheels (where they are more appropriate than lunches).

VOLUNTARY ORGANISATIONS AND SOCIAL CHANGE

While it was generally assumed that charities were properly associated with the provision of services, rather than with the advocacy which often tended to bring together groups of people who believed that human difficulties reflected flaws in the fabric of society as much as, if not more than, personal disabilities, there is now a growing recognition that these two elements are not mutually exclusive, and many organisations within the voluntary sector in general, as well as those working with old people in particular, have seen a powerful combination in using the information at their disposal as a tool for seeking to change attitudes or ultimately legislative provisions.

Thanks to an understanding and increasingly liberal view on the part of the Charity Commissioners, the growth of this element associated with the function of pressure groups has been widespread, so that very few charities would now shy away from playing at least some part in the process of social reform. Age Concern England now provides a Research Assistant for the All Party Pensioner Group in Parliament. It was the first major voluntary organisation enjoying charitable status to make such a move with the explicit approval of the Charity Commissioners. It was felt that constitutional commitments to follow the classic headings of charity in seeking to abolish poverty, to enhance health, to extend education, could sometimes be better fulfilled by government action than by providing palliatives for individual sufferers.

A mixture of advocacy and the provision of services on a mutual-aid basis has been a crucial feature of the growing movement of retired people themselves, following in the tradition of the many self-help movements of the nineteenth century. While even the largest organisations of retired people in the United Kingdom are minute in comparison with those in many other countries, and particularly in the United States, they have increasingly become one of the mechanisms through which older people themselves are able to find expression.

Table 8.1 Personal services to the individual at home

Aids to the infirm, sick and handicapped
Assistance with the administration of local trust funds
Day and night sitter-in services
Diversional occupations for handicapped
Emergency supplies of fuel, furniture and bedding
Escort services
Gardening
Hair washing, shaving, bathing, foot care
Help in the home
Home nursing requisites (loan or provision of)
House decorating and repairs
Housing problems of the elderly or disabled
Library (mobile or special facilities)
Meals-on-wheels
Nursing aid service (including simpler personal services, blanket bathing, etc.)
Outings and entertainments
Prevention of accidents
Provision of clothing, in recommended cases
Reading
Shopping, collecting prescriptions and pensions
Tape recordings for the housebound (church services, messages from relatives, etc.)
Transport (by cars and specially adapted vehicles)
Travelling companions (to aged or infirm needing to make a journey)
Visiting housebound and others in need of help
Wireless and TV sets (provision and/or repairs)

Table 8.2 Community services outside the home

After-care and rehabilitation
Boarding out of old people
Chiropody — nail-cutting
Courses for the elderly
Diversional occupations and trolley shops in local authority homes and voluntary homes
Emergency (e.g. floods, fire), general help
Entertainments
Handicraft and other classes
Health education
Help in local authority and voluntary homes (particularly at times of staff shortage or illness)
Holidays (groups and individuals)
Hospital car service
Job-finding schemes
Lunch clubs
Residential homes and hostels
Short-stay homes (including convalescent beds and to relieve relatives)
Social and recreational clubs
Training and occupational centres (assistance in)
Welfare foods (distribution of)
Workshops and sheltered employment schemes

General:
  Advice and information
  Education and research
  Publicity for available services
  Training courses and conferences for voluntary workers

Even setting aside the population differences between Great Britain and the United States, there is nothing on this side of the Atlantic to compare with the massive white collar American Association of Retired People, with over twenty million members, and the trade-union-based National Senior Citizens movement, with chapters throughout the country. But even though smaller and still lacking the power of the American pensioner movement, with its influence on the social and political life of the United States, increasing numbers of retirement organisations, often associated with occupational groupings or a common former employer, are beginning to illustrate how older people can both say things together about the policies they would like to see introduced, and do things together in terms of helping each other with practical tasks, offering a framework for social activities and providing sympathetic care during periods of distress.

In broad terms, the voluntary and charitable sector as a provider of services or advocate will have been seen to encompass direct service provision by those who may not be old, to self-help groups involving older people themselves. The other feature of the more traditional role for charitable organisations which has diminished considerably in recent years with the advent of the Welfare State, but is still a major force, lies in the provision of residential care or income support to replace or augment occupational pensions, private means or social security benefits.

Here there are a wide range of charitable organisations, many of which are associated with trade or professional benevolent institutions, where long-standing endowments, fund-raising events or subscriptions from members who are still economically active provide gifts for those who qualify for benevolent support under the terms of their rules and regulations. In this context, the term 'qualification' may mean either or both a level of age, infirmity or poverty and a relationship with the particular group in question so that, for example, beneficiaries must be ex-servicemen to qualify for charities associated with the Armed Forces, or retired gardeners, publicans or governesses to be eligible for help from charities which specify their former occupational requirements.

THE FUTURE FOR VOLUNTARY ORGANISATIONS

Although the societies, which may well be old-established organisations, concentrate on limited financial support or on providing sheltered housing and residential care, a number are beginning to look to the future in a less restricted way. For instance, the charitable agency with (say) two residential establishments, in perhaps the north and south of the country, is too distant from the homes of many potential beneficiaries, for whom the advantages of secure care may not outweigh an understandable preference for remaining in their own homes with support, or at least in the areas where they have lived for much of their lives. In this respect, as in so many others, the voluntary and charitable sector is having to look seriously at ways in which it can best deploy its resources in the remaining decades of the century. Undoubtedly one key to the future, as in the public sector, is to concentrate on providing individual responses to particular people, whose circumstances will differ even from those with superficial similarities, in specially designed packages of care rather than in establishing services or general systems of distributing help in cash, in kind or in service without first testing its relevance to the old person on the receiving end.

In this respect, the traditional and often quoted virtue of flexibility on the part of the voluntary sector, and its capacity to innovate, will be fully tested in the years to come. In the final analysis, its lack of bureaucratic restraints and what should be its commitment to excellence should remain central features of its administration.

REFERENCES

Anon. (1909). Report of Royal Commission on the Poor Laws and Relief of Distress
Anon. (1952). Report of the Committee on the Law and Practice Relating to Charitable Trusts. HMSO, London
Anon. (1968). Report of the Committee on Local Authority and Allied Social Services. HMSO, London
Anon. (1969). Report on the Voluntary Worker in the Social Services. Allen and Unwin, London
Beveridge, W. (1948). *Voluntary Action*. A report on methods of social advance. Allen and Unwin, London
Hobman, D. B. (1965). *A Guide to Voluntary Service*. HMSO, London

9

The Role of the General Practitioner and the Primary Health Care Team

Charles Freer and Idris Williams

INTRODUCTION

Most medical and nearly all social care for old people now takes place in the community. Historically, society's response to the care of the poor, the infirm and the mentally ill was to institutionalise. For humane and economic reasons, the emphasis is now on care in the community, and under the pressure of a growing elderly population this has become national policy. Indeed, the present situation is that care should not only be in the community, but should also be provided by the community. Thus, the role of the family and friends is seen as crucial in providing basic care with State services supplementing this when necessary, sometimes as a last resort. This policy has implications for those providing both medical and social services in the community. This chapter presents a general practitioner view of the implications for primary health care services, and after a brief descriptive introduction will consider some of the challenges and changes evident in the delivery of primary medical care.

GENERAL PRACTITIONER CARE OF OLDER PEOPLE

In the United Kingdom the medical care of older people in the community is provided by the general practitioner. He has a list of patients, the average number being around 2000, of which 15 per cent will be over 65 and 6 per cent over 75 years of age. There is wide variation in both list size and the proportion of elderly, with some south coast practices having as many as 45 per cent of their patients over 65 years. General practitioner services are administered by Family Practitioner Committees, and the general practitioner (unlike hospital doctors) is not salaried but contracted to provide services for patients on his 'list'. He is paid by a complicated system of capitation, item of service and basic practice allowance. The extra work involved in caring for elderly patients is recognised by an increase in capitation fee for the over-65s and a further increase for the over-75s. Every person has access to the general practitioner with whom he or she is registered; cover is provided on a 24 hours per day basis every day of the year. The general practitioner must provide a deputy when he is not available; this is done either by arrangement with partners or through deputising services.

There is an absence of good detailed information on the work of general practitioners with older people, but a study of 90 000 patient consultations, 18 000 of which were with patients over 65, has shown interesting variations in patterns of work between general practitioners and between different age groups of patients (Wilkin and Williams, 1986). Not surprisingly, general practitioners were involved in more follow-up with their elderly patients, and made more home visits and referrals to nursing and social services for older as compared with younger patients. Elderly patients appear to be investigated less than younger patients, but referral rates to hospital clinics did now show any relationship to the age of patients. However, within these overall rates, considerable variation was found between doctors in the patterns of care provided for older patients. The mean referral rate to consultants for patients over 65 was 6 per cent of all consultations for all the doctors in the study, but 13 per cent had rates of more than 10 per 100 consultations and an equal proportion had rates of less than 2 per 100 consultations. These differences were not related to differences in the availability of hospital services for the elderly in different parts of the study area. Surprisingly, the proportion of elderly patients on the list of a general practitioner did not show any significant effect on his overall workload. The variation described does not necessarily reflect varying standards of care. It might simply reflect different interpretations of what is appropriate, or different perceptions of the role of the general practitioner and of the other professions and agencies working in the primary care arena.

CHANGES IN GENERAL PRACTICE

Until about thirty years ago the prevailing model of general practice was a single-handed doctor working alone, without an appointment system or paramedical staff, from a small converted shop. Since then, there have been dramatic changes, encouraged by incentives for group practice, partial reimbursement of ancillary staff salaries, the attachment of district nurses and health visitors, the building of health centres and financial aid for the construction of custom-built premises. At the same time, the emergence of vocational training for general practice (now a compulsory requirement for entry), the influence of the Royal College of General Practitioners and the establishment of departments of general practice in most British medical schools has led to much thought and discussion about the role of general practitioners in contemporary society. This professional growth has created a climate of change and a desire to examine the standards and quality of care. The elderly have not received a high priority in this context, but the principles of care listed in Table 9.1 are extracted from a report on the potential contribution of family doctors to the primary care of older people (Almind *et al.*, 1983).

Table 9.1   Principles of good primary care of the elderly (adapted from Almind *et al.*, 1983)

1. To help elderly people prevent unnecessary loss of function.

2. To help elderly people prevent and treat health problems which adversely affect quality of life in old age.

3. To supplement the care given by neighbours and friends and try to prevent the breakdown of informal support systems.

4. To help elderly people have a good death as well as a good life.

Of course, such principles are the ideal and are, as such, aims rather than objectives; but it is important and useful to examine some of the reasons why such principles can be hard to achieve in day-to-day practice.

CONSTRAINTS TO 'GOOD' PRIMARY GERIATRIC CARE

The Organisation of Primary Care Services

The administrative arrangements for primary care are complex and the result of historical evolution rather than any logical planning. The Family Practitioner Committee is responsible for medical services through contracts with general practitioners (who are in essence self-employed) and also administer dental, ophthalmological and pharmaceutical services. The District Health Authority is responsible for district nursing, health visiting, and sometimes domiciliary physiotherapy, occupational speech therapy, occupational therapy and chiropody. Special nursing liaison schemes involving hospitals are also administered through the Health Authority. Community social services are administered by local authorities through their Social Services Committees. They are responsible for a wide range of activities, and those particularly relevant to the elderly include home helps, meals-on-wheels, luncheon clubs, aids and appliances, and short- and long-term accommodation. The areas served by these three administrative bodies are rarely coterminous, and developing policies and plans at the team level can be difficult, if not impossible, because individual members have to relate to different employers, or are subject to constraints and policies at a higher administrative level.

It is also important to recognise that although the work of the general practitioner has changed dramatically in a very short period of time, the 'independent contractor' status is still highly valued by many and can make it difficult to develop a genuine team approach.

Motivation

Sociologists have long recognised that different illnesses have different degrees of status, and contemporary medical courses still reflect an adherence to a disease model with an emphasis on investigation and surgical or pharmacological management. It is, therefore, not surprising that many medical graduates do not view the health problems of the elderly as the most exciting of challenges — despite the enormous advances in assessment and management that have been developed through the rapid growth of geriatric medicine.

Education and Training

Since the Report of the Royal Commission on Medical Education (1968), medical schools have attempted to expand the disease model to include a social and psychological dimension, but much still needs to be done to achieve a truly integrated curriculum rather than adding behavioural science courses to what in most medical schools remains a predominantly bio-medical course. Diminishing negative stereotypes and preconceived notions about older people and their problems will be no more easy with doctors than with the rest of the population. It is likely, however, that many young doctors would respond to a greater emphasis on the clinical skills that can be successfully applied to many of the health problems experienced by older people, but this will only occur if the content and recent advances in geriatric medicine have a much larger place in the vocational training of general practitioners.

Demand-led Service

A large proportion of the work of general practitioners involves responding to health problems recognised and presented by patients. This is often seen as a weakness, relying, as it does, on the patient, and it is widely accepted in general practice that more preventive and anticipatory services should be developed. Anticipatory care will be discussed in more detail later, but we shall see that the self-reporting skills of patients have perhaps been underestimated and it has to be said that most of the health problems seen by general practitioners are legitimate, someone needs to deal with them, and if preventive services were enlarged to any great extent, then this might diminish the availability of resources for patients presenting with problems.

General Practitioner Workload

The average duration of GP consultations is 5–7 minutes. This has been a source of constant debate among and about general practitioners, and in particular about the implications for 'good practice' and list size (Wilkin and Metcalfe, 1984; Morrell *et al.*, 1986; Morrell and Roland, 1987). It should be remembered that these are average figures and that, when necessary, consultations can last very much longer; it is also fair to say that for many of the problems seen in general practice, short consultations like 5 minutes are perfectly adequate. It is also true that for some elderly persons access to general practitioner services can be difficult. Geographical and telephone access is not always easy for the elderly, and appointment systems and reception areas can present daunting barriers. In addition, although many general practitioners are happy to make extra time available for older people, the atmosphere of busy waiting rooms, appointment buzzers and lights, etc., can all inhibit the older patient. The growth of group practice, deputising services and the shift away from routine follow-up home visits have all diminished the 'personal doctoring' style which is particularly appreciated by many, but especially by older patients.

Expectations of the Elderly Patient

These barriers to general practitioner care are often compounded by the elderly person's own negative stereotyping. Many see their health problems as being the inevitable consequence of ageing, and perhaps the most constant feature of the older patient is the apology 'for bothering the busy doctor'. For older people who spent their formative years before the introduction of the Welfare State, this was perhaps not surprising, and there was a general feeling and prediction that this might change for individuals more accustomed to the free access of the National Health Service. As yet, no real evidence for this has emerged, and those working with older people still find that most are reluctant to make significant demands on the system.

These barriers to improved health care for older people are of concern but do not justify an overly pessimistic view of services; nor should they obscure the significant changes and improvements that have occurred since the introduction of the National Health Service in 1948. These improvements continue, and the remainder of this chapter will consider some of the important areas where debate and movement are most likely to occur.

CURRENT AND FUTURE CHANGES

The Organisation of Primary Health Care Services

Meeting the health needs of a growing elderly population will require attention to the overall structure of primary health care services and how these services are delivered at the team level. 1986 witnessed the publication of two relevant documents — the Government Green Paper on primary health care (Secretary of State for Social Services, 1986) and the Cumberlege Report on community nursing services (Department of Health and Social Security, 1986). There seems little doubt that the complex and unwieldy administrative structures would benefit from changes in attitude and perhaps legislation that would allow for a more creative mix of services that can be tailored for local and rapidly changing needs. The Green Paper was disappointing in that it failed to include some of the anticipated suggestions about local primary care franchises and other ways to experiment with primary health care. In contrast, the Cumberlege Report included proposals for geographic nurse attachment which met with an angry response from many general practitioners. It is unlikely that change will ever occur unless new and challenging proposals are put up for consideration. Sadly, it seems that the very comprehensive nature of the National Health Service makes local experimentation extremely difficult, whereas in countries such as the United States, where health services are pluralistic and patchy, many more innovative schemes have been introduced and tested.

Primary Health Care Team

Further changes are likely to occur in the team process, including the possible creation of new health professionals with a particular responsibility for the elderly.

Current trends in the way primary health care teams operate reflect a more complex yet realistic approach to the day-to-day conditions and demands of primary care than earlier more simple models. The main members of the team are the district nurse, health visitor, general practitioner, practice nurse and midwife. This can be called the macro-team. Beyond these individuals is a wider network which includes practice reception and secretarial staff, physiotherapists, occupational therapists, speech therapists, chiropodists, pharmacists, priests and many others. These can be called the mega-team. In practice, usually one team member from either the mega- or macro-team identifies a need. A small number of others then become involved because of their specific expertise and contribute to the solution. This small unit can be called the mini-team. It dissolves when the need is met, leaving only the key members to continue care. An example might be an old lady who slips on the ice and injures her arm. The general practitioner deals with the bruising and grazing, but the expertise of the district nurse and the health visitor or social worker is needed: one to arrange the dressings, and the other, social help to assist with cooking and housework. As the patient recovers, the mini-team will become less involved but the health visitor or social worker will continue to monitor functional status.

The changing roles of district nurses and health visitors with regard to the care of the elderly and the development of community nurses specialising in this age group are discussed in some detail in the next chapter. The development of nurse practitioners (nurses with additional training in diagnostic skills and with permission to prescribe medicines) has been receiving renewed attention, and, again, it is possible that geriatric nurse practitioners could fulfil an important role in the primary care team. However, before any additional health workers are added to what is already an expensive and labour-intensive service, it will be necessary to establish that existing team members are being used appropriately and efficiently.

Standards of General Practitioner Care

The early 1980s witnessed a renewed concentration on the type of care being offered, and a major impetus has come from the Royal College of General Practitioners' policy statement on quality in general practice (1985). This theme is also reflected in the Government's Green Paper on primary care (Secretary of State for Social Services, 1986), which proposes a 'good practice' allowance. Many general practitioners doubt whether such a reward mechanism is feasible, but at the same time there is a growing climate of support for finding ways to improve and reward standards of care. Age Concern have shown considerable interest in this with regard to their client group, and their report on practice guidelines (1986) offers a framework for examining the quality of primary care for older patients.

Augmented Home Care

To succeed in keeping older people in their own homes as long as possible may require not simply an increase in resources, but also changes in the way existing and possibly new resources are used. One illustration of this which has received surprisingly little publicity and attention is what has been described as 'augmented home care' (Currie *et al.*, 1980; Gibbins *et al.*, 1982). The essential feature of this model is that older people who have an acute problem or crisis and would probably be admitted for institutional care are seen quickly for a multidisciplinary assessment, and whatever resources are required to maintain the individual in his or her own home are provided without delay. The key to the system is that the organisers of the scheme are able to mobilise whatever health and social service resources are required and provide them at the level needed to maintain the person in his or her own home. This may not require additional resources, but may require existing health and social service staff to be involved in a way that is different from their usual practice. For example, district nurses may be required to spend an entire shift in the patient's home rather than a daily or twice-daily visit, or the general practitioner may be required to make three or four daily visits to the patient's home. An unpublished example of this in Lewisham used joint funding to employ a small number of additional personnel, to allow staff to be used in this intensive fashion. The limited amount of work that has been done in this field suggests that a significant number of patients who would otherwise have been institutionalised have been allowed to remain in their own homes, with accompanying cost savings. Experiments like this have been all too rare in Britain, but it is hoped that future years will see further examples and perhaps even the results of these isolated trials leading to more widespread changes in the use of primary care resources.

Preventive and Anticipatory Care

The belief that disease should be sought at an asymptomatic stage has been popular since the early 1960s, but after thirty years of geriatric screening no clear evidence of medical or economic benefit has emerged (Freer, 1985). Perhaps just as well, since the cost of regular surveillance of all older people would be enormous. Selective screening of high-risk groups would be attractive but as yet no practical strategies for doing this have emerged (Taylor *et al.*, 1983). Current attention has focused on two other approaches — one, the use of a two-stage process beginning with an initial screening letter; and the other, based on the knowledge that 90 per cent of all over-75-year-olds see their general practitioner at least once a year, adding a brief anticipatory assessment to the routine contact. Various trials of these approaches are being conducted in several centres (Taylor and Buckley, 1987). Concentrating on those elderly seen by doctors might raise concern about infrequent or non-attending patients; but several studies have now shown that the self-reporting of elderly patients is very appropriate and that older people not seen for over a year by their general practitioners are, in general, fit and healthy (Ebrahim *et al.*, 1984; Williams, 1984; Williams and Barley, 1985). It is likely that opportunistic screening or case-finding will undergo significant development over the next few years.

Links between Primary Care and Informal Carers

Several sections in this book draw attention to the vital contribution made by relatives and other informal carers. Recognition of this support, and also the enormous stress on informal supporters, has concentrated more attention on 'caring for the carers'. What has received less attention has been improving communication between the formal and informal networks — i.e. including informal carers in the mega-team. No doubt, in many individual situations relatives are able to communicate freely and appropriately with nurses or general practitioners, but there is a need for systematic attempts to develop guidelines and educational material which would allow older patients and their relatives to have a more detailed idea of services available, and how and when to request them. Not only does better communication make sense, but also the onus of responsibility cannot always lie with members of the primary health care team. Self-care has always made a significant contribution in this and other age groups, and informed self-reporting would help to shift the doctor–patient relationship from the traditional and often paternalistic model to one in which the patient and relatives have a more equal partnership.

The Use of Volunteers

Over the last century, informal care has frequently developed into more formal volunteer services and, indeed, some of these — for example, district nursing and meals-on-wheels — have been absorbed into health and social services. There is renewed interest in the potential of volunteers, and the elderly are an obvious target group. At the same time, with a growing retired population the many fit elderly are an important source of volunteers.

There is likely to be continued expansion of volunteer services at the grassroots level, but in his chapter David Hobman discusses the possible conflicts with trade unions, and at a time of high unemployment developments may well be a source of controversy. It is also important to appreciate that no services are ever totally cost-free. Training and administration are as important to volunteer activities as to formal services, and these costs can be substantial.

Institutional Care in the Community

There is general agreement that patients being admitted to private residential and nursing homes, especially those who are receiving State support, should receive a pre-admission assessment. However, this time-consuming process requires a degree of clinical expertise, and there has been much less agreement on how this should be done, who should pay for it and who should do it. The general practitioner may have some part to play in this process and would certainly be in a position to have some detailed multidimensional knowledge about the patient. Until the logistics and costings of this exercise can be agreed, the prevailing situation where Social Services have the main responsibility for assessment is likely to continue.

The rapid development of private homes, particularly in some semirural areas, has meant a steep increase in the number of dependent elderly patients on the lists of some general practitioners. This situation can create extreme difficulties for some doctors, and means that these patients do not receive the level of medical care that they require. It is likely that this situation will receive urgent attention at both local and national levels.

CONCLUSION

Primary care is demanding work. Dealing with a wide spectrum of ill-health and all age groups is a challenging, but often frustrating task; not least with the problems of the elderly, which are often multiple, complex and surrounding by an overwhelming sense of hopelessness or finality that can affect all involved.

In any human system there are bound to be deficiencies, and it is perhaps too easy to be critical. Overall, the changes in primary care in recent years have been impressive, reflecting a general increased awareness of the particular health needs of the elderly and many examples of attempts to turn good intentions into good practice.

Space has dictated only a cursory examination of the topics included in this chapter. However, it is hoped that it has given an indication of some of the more important areas where further development can be expected. There are grounds for optimism, and it is to be hoped that existing deficiencies, rather than leading to self-criticism and low morale, will be seen as a challenge for the future.

REFERENCES

Age Concern (1986). *Meeting the Needs of Older People. Some Practice Guidelines.* Age Concern England, Mitcham

Almind, G., Freer, C. B., Gray, J. A. M. and Warshaw, G. (1983). *The Contribution of the Primary Care Doctor to the Medical Care of the Elderly in the Community* (A report from the Kellogg International Scholarship Program on Health and Aging). Institute of Gerontology, University of Michigan, Ann Arbor

Currie, C., Smith, R. and Williamson, J. (1980). A scheme of augmented home care for the acutely and sub-acutely ill elderly patient: A report on a pilot study. *Age and Ageing*, **9**, 173

Department of Health and Social Security (1986). *Neighbourhood Nursing: A Focus for Care* (The Cumberlege Report). HMSO, London

Ebrahim, S., Hedley, R. and Sheldon, M. (1984). Low levels of ill health among elderly non-consulters in general practice. *Br. Med. J.*, **289**, 1273

Freer, C. B. (1985). Geriatric screening: a reappraisal of preventive strategies in the care of the elderly. *J. Roy. Coll. Gen. Pract.*, **35**, 288

Gibbins, F., Lee, M., Davison, P. R., O'Sullivan, P., Hutchinson, M. and Murphy, D. R. (1982). Augmented home nursing as an alternative to hospital care for chronic elderly invalids. *Br. Med. J.*, **284**, 330

Morrell, D. C., Evans, M., Morris, R. and Roland, M. O. (1986). The 'five minute' consultation: effect of time constraint on clinical content and satisfaction. *Br. Med. J.*, **292**, 870

Morrell, D. C. and Roland, M. O. (1987). How can good general practice care be achieved? *Br. Med. J.*, **294**, 161

Report on the Royal Commission on Medical Education 1965–1968 (The Todd Report, 1968). Cmnd. 3569, HMSO, London

Royal College of General Practitioners (1985). *Quality in General Practice*. Policy Statement 2, London

Secretary of State for Social Services, Wales, Northern Ireland and Scotland (1986). *Primary Health Care: An Agenda for Discussion*. Cmnd. 9771, HMSO, London

Taylor, R. and Buckley, G. (Eds.) (1987). *Preventive Care of the Elderly: Review of Current Developments*. Occasional Paper No. 35, Royal College of General Practitioners, London

Taylor, R., Ford, G. and Barber, J. H. (1983). *The Elderly at Risk: A Critical Review of Problems in Screening and Case-finding*. Age Concern England, Mitcham

Wilkin, D. and Metcalfe, D. H. M. (1984). List size and patient contact in general medical practice. *Br. Med. J.*, **289**, 1501

Wilkin, D. and Williams, E. I. (1986). Pattern of care for the elderly in general practice. *J. Roy. Coll. Gen. Pract.*, **36**, 567

Williams, E. I. (1984). Characteristics of patients over 75 not seen during one year in general practice. *Br. Med. J.*, **288**, 119

Williams, E. S. and Barley, N. H. (1985). Old people not known to the general practitioner: low risk group. *Br. Med. J.*, **291**, 251

10

The Nurse's Role in Health Promotion and Preventive Health Care of the Elderly

Karen Luker

INTRODUCTION

The widespread attachment of district nurses and health visitors to general practitioners has created the opportunity for a team approach to primary health care, but how these teams are organised and the way individual members operate vary to a considerable degree. This lack of uniformity reflects a combination of factors, including different priorities on the part of the employing Health Authorities, variations between individual nurses in the interpretation of their role and the differing expectations and referral policies of others, especially general practitioners.

This chapter will examine the contribution nurses can make to the primary health care of the elderly, but first, to allow the nurse's involvement to be considered in the context of other professional and lay care, some results from a large-scale survey of the elderly in Manchester will be discussed.

SERVICES AND SUPPORT FOR THE ELDERLY

Over 1400 individuals aged over 65 years, a 3.76 per cent stratified random sample of the total elderly population of Trafford, Manchester, were interviewed (Luker and Perkins, 1987). The health visitor/client ratio in Trafford was 1:3000 and all were generic health visitors, with no nurses or others specialising in the care of the elderly. Fifty per cent of the study sample had visited the general practitioner in the three months before the interview. Table 10.1 shows the level of support provided by relatives for various tasks. This provides further evidence, if any is needed, for the importance of families in the support of elderly people. The results also

155

Table 10.1 Percentage of elderly individuals receiving assistance from spouse and daughter/
daughter-in-law for selected activities of daily living ($n = 1406$)

Activity	Spouse % (No.)	Daughter/daughter-in-law % (No.)
Light housework	51.0 (88)	21.6 (37)
Getting in or out of bath/shower	39.6 (44)	33.3 (37)
Extra washing because of incontinence	19.5 (16)	19.5 (16)

showed that professional services were more likely to be given to those without caring relatives; that is, there may be an implicit, if unstated, policy which entrenches family, especially female relatives, in the carer role. A further and related point raised by the results is that the distribution of resources should not be taken to reflect the pattern of need in the elderly population, since this will underestimate the number of very frail and failing elderly who are being maintained in the community by high levels of family support.

This latter situation not infrequently leads to sudden and crisis presentations to health and social services when the relatives become exhausted. It may be that some of these crises could be avoided if the carers were given more professional support at an earlier stage and, for example, some services such as home helps were available for the relatives and not just the elderly person.

Table 10.2 shows the number of visits made by professional carers in the four weeks prior to the interview period. Other services were used by only a very small number of individuals, with no more than 9 per cent (133) of the sample visiting a day centre and just 2.7 per cent (39) receiving meals-on-wheels or using a luncheon club.

Table 10.2 Distribution of visits to elderly individuals by professional carers in the month
prior to interview ($n = 1406$)

Professional service	% (No.)
District nursing	6.7 (96)
Health visiting	0.6 (9)
Chiropody	29.0 (402)
Home help	14.0 (199)

Table 10.2 underlines that, compared with other professional carers, district nurses and especially health visitors have a much lower contact rate with older people, and the remainder of this chapter will focus on the work of nurses in the community, concentrating particularly on the potential and perhaps changing contribution of each to the anticipatory care of the elderly. The organisation of community nursing services has come under closer

scrutiny in recent years and the Cumberlege Report (Department of Health and Social Security, 1986) has provided a challenging set of thoughts and proposals. Within this wider debate about the organisation of services there are some important and fundamental issues concerning the role of nurses working within the community which need to be addressed.

HEALTH VISITING

The health visitor is a registered nurse with either an obstetrics certificate or a midwifery qualification, who has undertaken a further year of full-time study at an institute of higher education. The main focus of the health visitor's course is on child development, social aspects of disease, and health education and promotion. Historically, the health visitor was a child visitor, but now she is expected to search out unreported health needs and provide an anticipatory service, especially for vulnerable groups (Council for the Education and Training of Health Visitors, 1977), and for many years has held a brief for the so-called well elderly. In most cases, health visitors have not given this group priority status, and instead work to the traditional model of visiting families with children under 5 years of age and organising and staffing clinics for well babies. Health visitors' statistics show that only 13 per cent of individuals visited are 65 years or older (Central Statistical Office, 1985), and, despite the increasing numbers of older patients in society, the proportion of elderly people visited by health visitors has not increased since 1976.

This low level of health visitor involvement with the elderly, even in areas where there is generous health visitor staffing, has several possible explanations.

First, local Health Authorities' policies may lay down specific guidelines about the frequency of the health visitor visits to the under-5s, and the level of case-load in this age group may simply leave little time for involvement with other age groups.

Second, the personal preference of the health visitor is likely to be critical and is probably the major influence on whether elderly people will receive visits or not (Luker, 1979). Many may simply have chosen health visiting because of the mother and child orientation.

A small study (Luker, 1978) sought to explore the opinions of health visitors about the elderly, and there appeared to be some agreement that the elderly were an 'at-risk' group who should receive some priority. But at the same time, the health visitors did not regard the elderly as part of their case-load in the same way as they did the children. The policy in the study area was to visit an elderly person after he or she had consulted a general practitioner, from whom most referrals came. When asked about a specialised health visiting service for the elderly, most considered that it would be a depressing job and that it would be difficult to find health visitors willing to do it. It was felt that if everyone over the age of 75 years was to be visited on a regular basis, then a considerable number of specialised health visitors would be needed, since visits to the elderly were believed to take much longer than visits to other age groups. A comment by one respondent, 'You just can't get away', summed it all up. Dingwall (1977), in his study of the social organisation of health visitor training, commented that student health visitors did not like visiting the elderly, because it took too long. Dingwall hypothesised that the reason they could not terminate the visit was because it had no structure. The students were not in control, and, to use his words, 'they did not have an agenda'. Hence, the client took over.

Dingwall's observations were confirmed in another study (Luker, 1978), which found that infants aged up to 6 months appeared to receive the most intensive and structured visiting, while contacts with the elderly were the most aimless and unstructured. It seemed that the developmental model underlying preventive child care and central to health visitor training provided this structure. It is likely that the absence of a similar model and structure for the elderly makes it difficult for many health visitors to deal easily with their problems.

A third factor in the health visitors' involvement with the elderly is the attitude and referral patterns of other professionals. The general practitioner is particularly important in this respect, and his referral behaviour will be influenced by both his attitude to the elderly and the value he places on the role of the health visitor. Wilkin and Metcalfe (1984) found that, during three weeks of data collection on the work of general practitioners, almost half made no referrals to nursing or health visiting services and 65 per cent no referrals to social services.

Whatever these obstacles, the pro-active role of health visiting, with its central commitment to health promotion, offers significant theoretical potential for anticipatory care of older people. Vetter and his colleagues (1986) have used their research findings to argue for the unique role of health visitors in promoting health in the elderly. Rethinking priorities is feasible within the context of the primary health care team, and health visitors could contribute far more to the care of the elderly than they do at present. It would seem reasonable to look to national organisations such as the Health Visitors' Association for these types of initiative. Yet the HVA's joint policy statement with the British Geriatrics Society (1986) failed to grasp the key issues which concern many health visitors in daily contact with the elderly. To acknowledge, as the report does, that health visiting services must become more responsive to the needs of the elderly without offering firm proposals as to how this could be done is disappointing and unhelpful. Of further concern was the report's suggestion that health visitors should make contact with *all* elderly people who fall within their area of responsibility. This universalistic approach to surveillance would require a massive increase in health visiting resources (Barber and Wallis, 1982) and is surely difficult to contemplate in the absence of any clear evidence of health or economic benefits from such a system (Freer, 1985).

The contribution that health visitors will come to make to the care of the elderly in the future will depend on national and local policies and local resources, but cannot be seriously debated or planned without reference to district nursing services.

DISTRICT NURSING

The district nurse is a registered nurse who has undergone a further period of training to prepare her to work in the community. Enrolled nurses may also train as district nurses, but they are responsible to a registered nurse. Since 1981, district nurse training has been mandatory and the syllabus has been extended to reflect the wide variety of work which district nurses undertake in the community. Currently, training is of twelve months' duration and takes place in institutes of higher education.

The location of her work is usually the home, although many district nurses run clinics in health centres and doctors' surgeries. They work almost entirely from referrals from other agencies, although most of the patients come from the general practitioner. Approximately 45 per cent of patients visited are over 65 years of age and 50 per cent are between the ages of 5 and 64 (Central Statistical Office, 1985). Since older patients are usually visited most frequently and the care that they require usually takes longer to provide than for younger patients, it is likely that the district nurse spends the majority of her time with the elderly. As can be seen from the Trafford figures, she certainly spends considerably more of her time with the elderly than do health visitors.

Historically, the emphasis in district nurse training was firmly placed on providing a reactive service giving direct care to individuals. In contrast, health visiting has concentrated on health promotion and health education with both individuals and groups. The Royal Commission on the National Health Service (Department of Health and Social Security, 1979) acknowledged the contribution that the district nurse makes to the care of the sick, but envisaged an expansion of this role to include health education to the elderly and other client groups. Recent district nurse training curricula reflect this shift in orientation. However, Hunt's study (1978) suggested that district nurses were reluctant to take a health education role. According to Phillipson (1983), this lack of enthusiasm is partly accounted for by district nurses not seeing health education and health promotion as part of nursing care. A distinction can be made here between informal and formal education. In their routine work, district nurses talk to patients and carers, and much of the content of these conversations could be classified as health education. It is likely that many district nurses see health education as a more formal process and thereby underestimate their existing involvement in health promotion. It is also likely that district nursing's commitment to direct care will inhibit the acceptance of a formal preventive role for district nurses. At the same time, some in health visiting may use this recent support for a greater involvement by district nurses in health education as justification for the lack of involvement with the elderly.

Clearly, these role and boundary issues need to be resolved with some degree of urgency if the elderly are not to be deprived of community nursing support. So what of the future?

FUTURE DIRECTIONS

The training of nurses working in both hospitals and the community will undergo major changes in the next twenty years. There are several possible developments which might affect community care of the elderly.

First, health visitors and district nurses may continue very much as at present, with neither group making any special commitment to the care of older people. This would probably necessitate the creation of an additional team member with special responsibility for older people. Indeed, some health districts already have health assistants who are appointed with sole responsibility for this age group. In the present financial climate, the creation of an additional health professional for the elderly would have to be evaluated carefully, and a sensible first step would be to assess the efficiency of current community nursing services.

Second, specialisation might occur within the health visiting role, with the emergence of a geriatric health visitor. Although there are already such positions in Britain, a more formal expansion of this is a distinct possibility and is very much in line with the community nurse specialist, as recommended in the Cumberlege Report (Department of Health and Social Security, 1986). There may be problems in attracting sufficient recruits from nursing to work with this age group. Any expansion of specialist health visitors and district nurses would probably mean that they could no longer be practice-attached but instead geographically based and thereby involved with a large number of general practitioners. This notion of a 'neighbourhood base' is again in keeping with the recommendations of the Cumberlege Report, and though many British general practitioners are opposed to this move, some Health Authorities may prefer to use their resources in this way.

Third, there has been renewed support for nurse practitioners — that is, nurses with additional training in diagnosis and treatment and possibly with permission to prescribe from a limited list — and this might pave the way for the emergence of geriatric nurse practitioners.

CONCLUSIONS

Community nursing has always made a vital and important contribution to primary health care. With growing numbers of very old people and the current policy to promote care in the community, the future role of nurses will become yet more crucial. Nurses and their representative bodies have shown that they are prepared to take the initiative in the present climate of change, but the elderly are a relatively powerless group in society, and, because they straddle professional boundaries, it is all the more important that nurses reaffirm their commitment to this group by positive action rather than by policy intent.

REFERENCES

Barber, J. H. and Wallis, J. B. (1982). The effects of a system of geriatric screening and assessment on general practice workload. *Hlth Bull.*, **40**, 125

Central Statistical Office (1985). *Social Trends, 15*. HMSO, London

Council for the Education and Training of Health Visitors (1977). *An Investigation into the Principles of Health Visitor Training*. Croom Helm, London

Department of Health and Social Security (1979). *Royal Commission on the National Health Service* (Chairman: Sir Alec Merrison). HMSO, London

Department of Health and Social Security (1986). *Neighbourhood Nursing: A Focus for Care* (The Cumberlege Report). HMSO, London

Dingwall, R. (1977). *The Social Organisation of Health Visitor Training*. Croom Helm, London

Freer, C. B. (1985). Geriatric screening: a reappraisal of preventive strategies in the care of the elderly. *J. Roy. Coll. Gen. Pract.*, **35**, 288

Health Visitors' Association and British Geriatrics Society (1986). *Health Visiting and the Aged: A Joint Policy Statement*. HVA, London

Hunt, A. (1978). *The Elderly at Home*. HMSO, London

Luker, K. A. (1978). Goal attainment: A possible model for assessing the work of the health visitor. *Nursing Times*, **74** (30), 1257

Luker, K. A. (1979) Health visiting and the elderly. *Midwife, Hlth Vis. Comm. Nurse*, **15** (11), 457

Luker, K. A. and Perkins, E. S. (1987). The elderly at home service, needs and provision. *J. Roy. Coll. Gen. Pract.* (in press)

Phillipson, C. (1983). *Health Education and the Elderly*. Unpublished paper, Department of Adult Education, Keele University

Vetter, N. J., Jones, D. A. and Victor, C. R. (1986). A health visitor affects the problems others do not reach. *Lancet*, **2**, 30

Wilkin, D. and Metcalfe, D. H. H. (1984). List size and patient contact in general medical practice. *Br. Med. J.*, **289**, 1501

11

New Horizons in Hospital-based Care

Peter Millard

A journey of a thousand miles starts with but a single step.
(Chinese proverb: I Ching)

INTRODUCTION

The choice not to spend money on the development of a better style of medical services for the aged is a choice to spend on other things. Spending, planning and even dreaming are simply matters of priorities. Kaplan (1983) comments that in the long run money only flows as our ethic permits it to flow.

To reach 'new horizons' one must be prepared to start the journey. In this chapter I examine some past suggestions, reflect on the present and conclude with the way I would like to see us go forward. The chapter is a 'personal view' spiced with references to others' work.

HISTORICAL PERSPECTIVE

Gerocome or Geriatrics

Through the centuries many doctors have seen the need for better medical services for the elderly. Writing in 1752, John Smith's 'earnest desire' was that doctors should study the 'gerocomical part of physick' (Smith, 1752). In 1803 in Paris doctors urged the development of gerocome — medicines des vieillards (Stearns, 1977). 'Gerocome' (literally old age, tending — the science of treatment of the aged) is etymologically correct. Nascher (1909), an American physician working with the chronic sick, coined the word 'geriatrics' — literally old, healer. The British Geriatrics Society adopted the word in the 1950s to improve its image. Curiously, geriatrics has now in some circles become a term of abuse.

Some consultants prefer to use 'physician in geriatric medicine' or 'consultant in clinical gerontology'. Others argue that geriatrics as a specialty should not exist (for example, Leonard, 1976) or should reintegrate with general medicine (for example, Royal College of Physicians, 1977). Debate usually focuses on the management of acute disease in old age, yet past demands for a separate specialty arose from doctors working in chronic care institutions. Special pleading came from physicians who by force of circumstances found themselves working in local authority institutions. There they witnessed medical neglect and from there arose their visions of a better world.

Marjory Warren's Hypothesis

Marjory Warren (1943), the mother of British geriatric medicine, expressed these wartime sentiments:

> If we are to maintain the right to call ourselves a great nation we must make provision in our scheme for all members of the community, old and young, sick and well, poor and rich, helpless and independent.

In the 1930s she had been given clinical responsibility for the chronic sick wards of a Greater London infirmary. There she found unmarried mothers and their babies, orphans, the destitute and senile bedridden patients all housed in the same ward. Within those wards she began diagnosis, classification and treatment. She established a specialty of medicine (Adams, 1961), with its emphasis on rehabilitating the sick.

In 1946 Warren described a special medical service called 'geriatrics'. The summary of her paper concluded:

- There should be a change of attitude on the part of the medical profession towards the care of the chronic sick. When this is established the change will be reflected in nursing and other hospital staff.
- A higher standard and a great deal more work is needed in the care of the chronic sick.
- The creation of a specialty of geriatrics would stimulate better work and initiate research.
- The chronic sick should be diagnosed and treated in special blocks of a general hospital set up and equipped for the purpose.
- Chronic aged sick should be admitted to homes only through hospital units. All homes for the chronic sick should be attached to hospital units to ensure follow-up work.

Medical Responsibility for the Chronic Sick

Warren (1943) placed her faith in medical leadership. Wilson (1972) and Kayser-Jones (1981), who compared a geriatric hospital in England with an

American nursing home, considered medical leadership essential. Grimley-Evans and Graham (1984) drew attention to the inherent difficulty of placing reliance on charismatic leadership, yet the change that took place in medical care of the chronic sick and the consequent development of geriatric medical services is a direct result of placing responsibility for the care of the chronic sick upon physicians. Historically that chore had been ignored. Even in the temples of Aesculapius in ancient Greece, the chronic sick were excluded — 'for their presence would not bolster the temple's reputation for cure' (Bettman, 1956). Rosen (1967) illustrated history by quoting a minute of a medical staff committee, written in 1808:

> Certain medical practitioners tended to refer to the Dundee Royal Infirmary patients far advanced in illness who had no prospect of recovery. These people were not regarded as 'proper objects' of the infirmary which was never intended as an almshouse or poorhouse.
> What opinions would the public form of the skill of the medical attendants in the house, if upon looking at the annual reports it should appear that the cases of death were to those of recovery as three to one?

Geriatric medicine did not arise from within the profession: there is no organ, system or special skill which justified its development. Leonard (1976), concluding that there was no medical justification for a separate specialty, disregarded the fact that the specialty exists because responsibility for the chronic sick was transferred.

Sick or Infirm

The change occurred not because of 'desire', but because of complaints: Means and Smith (1983) describe how the complaints which followed the discharge of 140 000 chronic sick from acute hospitals in England in the first two days of World War II led to an inquiry. Lord Amulree, a member of that inquiry, later to become first president of the British Geriatrics Society, speaking in the debate in the House of Lords in support of Warren's hypothesis, considered that if government tried artificially to separate the frail from the sick, they would eventually have difficulty.

However, because frail elderly people, made homeless by bombing, had managed well in seaside hotels, sole responsibility for the chronic sick was placed on Regional Hospital Boards, while the frail remained with local government (Means and Smith, 1983). The sick and the infirm were separated.

Somerville Hastings' (1951) article gives the definitions of the then Ministry of Health:

> *Sick* — and therefore properly the responsibility of the regional hospital board — patients requiring continued medical treatment also supervision and

nursing care. This would include very old people who, though not suffering from any particular disease, are confined to bed on account of extreme weakness.

Infirm — and therefore properly the responsibility of the local authority — persons who are normally able to get up and who could attend meals either in the dining room or in a nearby day room. This class would also include those who need a certain amount of help from the staff in dressing, toilet, or moving from room to room, and those who from time to time — for example, in bad weather — may need to spend a few days in bed.

The decision to separate was based on evidence that the 'chronic sick' could be rehabilitated, not on evidence that the aged could be treated.

Treating the Aged Sick

> Many of the disabilities formerly regarded as the irreversible effects of senescence have come to be recognised as due to specific disease processes that can be mitigated or effectively treated.
>
> (Arnold and Exton-Smith, 1962)

Few doctors now believe that old age, *per se*, is a cause of frailty: chronological age, for example, is no longer a bar to anaesthesia for cataract surgery, pacemaker, hip replacements and other procedures. Modern doctors are changing their attitudes to the aged.

In 1948 wards were full of bed-bound patients. All services had to be developed. Williamson (1979) notes the historical development of the specialty of geriatric medicine; Howell (1974) describes the origins of the British Geriatrics Society, which through its twice-yearly meetings acted as a central focus for the discussion of change; and Hall, in a chapter in this book, describes the achievements of the specialty.

Paper titles reflect pride in achievement: 'The Geriatric Department and the community: value of hospital treatment of the aged' (Arnold and Exton-Smith, 1962); 'Making hospital geriatrics work' (Hodkinson and Jeffreys, 1972); 'No apology for geriatrics' (O'Brien *et al.*, 1973); 'Geriatric medicine in Hull: a comprehensive service, (Bagnall *et al.*, 1977); 'To rehabilitate or to vegetate' (Millard, 1978); 'Developing an active service in Scunthorpe' (Das Gupta, 1980); 'Integration of geriatrics with general medical services in Newcastle' (Grimley-Evans, 1983).

> From its origins as a 'last resort' service for elderly patients who did not respond to treatment in the traditional specialties, geriatric medicine developed into a medical sub-specialty concerned with the clinical, preventive, remedial and social aspects of health and disease in elderly people.
>
> (Department of Health and Social Security, 1981)

Districts with a good geriatric service were considered to give a better service to the community (Exton-Smith and Millard, 1973).

Attitudes change. In the mid-1970s papers started to be published expressing a view that there was no need for a specialty of geriatric medicine. Leonard (1976) wrote 'Can geriatrics survive?' Cross, a medical student, joined in with 'Geriatric medicine — death and rebirth' (Cross, 1977). Wilson (1972), a consultant geriatrician, wrote 'Geriatrics at the crossroads' and expressed concern that there could be two standards of service. In 1977 the Royal College of Physicians published a working party report that recommended reintegration of general medical and geriatric services.

Whereas in 1946 Warren had dreams of a better world, the 1970s heralded the thoughts that the better world was too costly. The Department of Health and Social Security (1981), discussing how the country could cope with the problem of an ageing population, wrote: '. . . if the country can afford the improvement the specialty could keep up'.

Both changing medical practice and concern at cost encouraged changing attitudes (Graham, 1983). If the experimental National Health Service nursing homes are successful, then 'leadership' responsibility can be given to nurses for long-term care. The consultants in geriatric medicine will lose overall responsibility while retaining the decision to admit, and geriatric medical services can then reintegrate.

Thirty years after gerocome was recommended in France, ageing was included in theses and demands for the specialty ceased (Stearns, 1977). Now in France there are separate acute, medium and long-stay services. Is history repeating itself in Britain? Is it wise to abandon the specialty and give up medical responsibility for the long-term care of the aged sick?

STYLE OF SERVICE

In his chapter, Hall has described in some detail the various components of geriatric services and compared the age-related with the integrated approach. Development of services depends upon local initiative, the resources available and central government funding. Government's continuing commitment to its 1948 decision is shown by the presence of acute admission units, day hospitals, psychogeriatric services, local authority day centres, meals-on-wheels, home helps, residential homes, etc., which reflect the use made locally of centrally allocated resources.

In 1985 Brocklehurst and Andrews published a review of the style of practice in departments of geriatric medicine. There were six styles:

combined acute and rehabilitation with separate long-stay	37.5 per cent
separate acute/rehabilitation long-stay	21.1 per cent
combined acute, rehabilitation and long-stay	21.1 per cent
separate acute and combined rehabilitation/long stay	7.5 per cent
rehabilitation and long-stay	2.3 per cent
mixed general medicine and geriatric	7.0 per cent

What style is the best? No one knows. In the absence of measurement, there can only be opinions (Feldstein, 1963).

O'Brien *et al.* (1973) report how an age-related service, aged 65 and over, led to a fall in the proportion of 'chronic' beds in relation to acute. Das Gupta (1980) shows how new hospital development enabled him to develop an age-related admission service which solved the problem of 'blocked beds' and resulted in the disappearance of a waiting list.

Hodkinson and Jeffreys (1972) have reported the development of an active service admitting 6.6 patients per bed per year. They considered that an essential difference between low and high turnover units is the absence of a waiting list, and a bed provision of less than the Department of Health and Social Security norm of 10 beds per 1000 persons over 65. They claimed that waiting lists blunt therapeutic effectiveness, cause deterioration to occur while patients await admission, decrease morale in hospital, and cause resistance to discharge and premature referral for admission.

Resources influence attitudes. I reported nursing male and female patients together (Millard, 1978) and increased turnover when the location and use of hospital beds was changed. Grimley-Evans (1983), on the basis of his experience in Newcastle, advocates an integrated model wherein general medicine and geriatric medicine share acute wards. The Royal College of Physicians (1977) encourages this approach, and tacit approval is given by the Department of Health and Social Security (1981) and by Irvine (1984). Wilson (1972) sees reintegration as a threat, since the elderly would lose the benefit of a committed team.

Services are also developed because of a perceived need. Feldstein (1963) considers that thinking in terms of 'need' is wrong. 'Need' is a misguided conception; planning should be based upon 'operational models', with decisions only being made after consideration of those factors that maximise or minimise equations in the model — failing that, decisions are made on feelings. It is no use asking the opinion of people who have no experience, for people who have no experience can have no opinion.

When change occurs, its outcome is unpredictable. One can only start from where one is; what is present influences the outcome. The effect varies. Some people visit the innovator, to return home and modify their work to suit their circumstances. Others hear first-hand, or second-hand, and like Chinese whispers the end result differs from the initial concept.

MEDICAL RESPONSIBILITY, NOT INTEREST

Responsibility for long-term care, not interest in long-term care, is the key. I am interested in improving care in my wards because I feel responsible. Indirectly I hope that my activities will improve services elsewhere. I am interested to see whether that happens — I am not responsible for seeing that it does.

I am concerned when patients admitted to my beds have obviously been misdiagnosed or mismanaged. I recognise that I am aware of such misdiagnosis and mismanagement because of my acquired knowledge. Wishing to reduce the level of my own mismanagement, I consider that research and study is beneficial. I do not know what system is best, but I recognise that if physicians are removed, then medical research ceases.

SPECIAL UNITS FOR THE AGED

Special units for the aged are essential. The *Encyclopaedia Britannica* 1911 edition lists many different types of specialist hospitals — cancer hospitals, hospitals for consumption, children's hospitals, cottage hospitals, ear, throat and nose hospitals, fever hospitals, maternity and lying-in hospitals, mental hospitals, ophthalmic hospitals, orthopaedic hospitals, paralysis and epileptic hospitals, skin and phototherapy hospitals, women's hospitals — but there is no mention of the aged. The plans for a 'hospital city' which foretell the present large district general hospitals exclude the aged and the chronic sick. They were not included in the plan, not because they did not exist, but because they were out of sight, out of mind, in local authority institutions. Hospital services for the elderly will only continue to develop if awareness is maintained of this group's priority status.

THE FUTURE

Thom (1975), a French professor of mathematics, contributed a monograph outlining the theoretical concept of model-making. His mathematical model will eventually allow prediction to be made after examinations of equations, but, as yet, we gaze into crystal balls: there are many opinions, few facts and no models. The future depends on the present. Choices are being made — even the choice to do nothing is a choice not to do something (Feldstein, 1963).

A fundamental principle of model-making is that one should make a temporal map — the inverse of that map then yields the logical succession. Examination of what has happened thus enables us to foresee what could happen. However, our present system is under pressure, and when that condition appertains, the succession may no longer be logical. A plastic cup, when pressed, first deforms and then breaks — the pattern of its breaking cannot be predicted; all we can predict is that the remnants will contain pieces of the cup.

Basic Principles

Pfeiffer (1985) has outlined some basic principles.

- Older patients are treatable.
- Care of the elderly requires a multidisciplinary approach.
- Intervention in the life of an older patient should always be preceded by a comprehensive assessment of that patient's overall functioning.
- Care of the elderly patient requires a new type of service: co-ordination of services or case management.
- The role of the family is critically important in the care of the older patient.
- Care of the elderly requires a special training in geriatrics and gerontology.
- Not only are older patients treatable; they are also teachable.
- Older patients are not only treatable and teachable; they also teach us about ageing.

Accepting Pfeiffer's principles, one can then apply those principles to the present pattern of services and use the temporal map to see what type of service will be present in the future.

Hospital Beds

The population is ageing. The stock of hospital beds is being reduced: a 20 per cent reduction in total bed stock and a 2 per cent reduction in beds allocated to geriatric medicine has occurred since 1948 (Millard, 1984). While the number of hospital beds within the National Health Service has declined, the number of beds in private hospitals has increased. The logical succession is that the National Health Service bed numbers will continue to decrease and the private sector hospital bed numbers will continue to increase.

Private medicine in the United Kingdom mainly deals with illness within the insured working population. The future task is therefore to provide hospital care for the aged population with a declining stock of National Health Service beds.

This policy is not based on recognition of the basic principle that elderly people are treatable, but assumes that treatment at all ages can be speeded up. Yet Vere (1983) states that productivity in acute hospitals will only be speeded up if weekends are abolished. The length of stay of aged people is longer than the length of stay of young people. Reliance on home helps for those who live alone often means discharge on a Monday or Tuesday. Bank holidays and statutory days off slow down productivity.

With an ageing population, it is probably impossible to speed up treatment indefinitely. Accepting that we wish to retain hospitals, then there must be a finite number of beds which each health district should provide.

Observation

If speed of treatment of the aged is a rate-limiting factor, and if elderly people need a different environment within the finite bed allocation, it would seem logical to develop special units for the aged in all district general hospitals.

Institutional Places

At the same time as the National Health Service hospital bed stock has declined, places in residential homes have increased by 250 per cent. The number of people deemed to require long-term care in hospital is decreasing; the number requiring nursing care in residential homes is increasing. The residential hotel is becoming a nursing home (Thompson, 1983).

The logical succession is that the number of hospital beds will continue to decrease and the number of places in care will continue to increase. In the United Kingdom in 1987, the expansion of care is no longer in the hospital or local authority sectors, but is seen in the private sector. Such care is seen to be cheaper; yet the most expensive patient is the one who never goes home.

The policy of expanding residential and nursing care as a solution to the problem of old age is in direct contrast to the policies operating in the hospital, and the underlying assumption must, therefore, be that the first basic principle expressed by Pfeiffer — that the older patient is treatable — is not accepted.

Observation

If treatment of the aged is possible, then a wiser way forward would be to experiment with reducing dependency in institutional care by introducing modern methods of treatment and a multidisciplinary approach.

Admission to Hospital

Fifteen per cent of the population aged 65 and over are admitted to hospital each year. The population is ageing, and thus the number requiring admission will increase. Requests for acute admission arise from doctors who are treating patients at home, in residential homes, in nursing homes and in long-stay wards. Illness, like random hits, knows no boundaries.

Policies of increasing numbers of places in sheltered housing, residential homes and nursing homes will have no influence on the random hit of illness. The presence of these units, while they are expanding in number, may make it easier to discharge people, but in stable state they can have no influence on acute admission numbers, nor can they make it easier to solve the problem of bed-blocking by transferring patients elsewhere.

A wiser policy would be to introduce a rationing system of expensive long-term care whereby admission to permanent care only took place after a thorough review by the multidisciplinary team which specialises in the care of the dependent elderly.

Observation

Expanding care in institutions as a means of caring can only be beneficial to the hospital service while that care is expanding — i.e. so long as the number of places is increasing. When that position appertains, discharge can be made to another place. As soon as the beds or community care places are full, then such policies exert no influence, for the vacancy rate then comes to equal the death/admission rate.

A wiser policy would be to use the resources being spent on care to expand treatment of the aged in all district general hospitals, for the hospital with its modern methods of diagnosis and treatment is the community's safety net.

A WAY FORWARD

In this personal review I have not touched on the subjects of teaching and research into the causes of dementia, confusion, immobility, falling, incontinence, contractures and pressure sores, but I believe that if physicians were allowed to give up responsibility for long-term care, the majority of research into the causes of these ailments would cease.

My basic principles would be:

- Medical responsibility for local authority residential homes should be transferred to the hospital service.
- No one should be admitted to a local authority home or to a government-funded place in a private or voluntary home without prior in-patient assessment in the beds of the Department of Geriatric Medicine, in the district general hospital.

- In those 42 health districts where there are no beds allocated to the Department of Geriatric Medicine in the district general hospital, those beds should be provided as a matter of urgency.
- All who are permanently accommodated in a long-term institution should have the right to be tended in single rooms with *en suite* washing and toilet facilities. All long-term residents should be able to keep personal belongings in their rooms.
- Named consultants should have contractual responsibility for the standard of medicine and care in long-term care wards and residential homes. Whether there should be separate age-related or integrated services of geriatric medicine should be decided after study of the resources available in each health district. These systems are expressions of local resource allocation, and the adoption of the type has resource implications.

CONCLUSION

In this overview I have concentrated on the hospital, because the hospital is the ultimate community safety net. Policies that ignore what happens within the hospital will, in my view, be less likely to succeed. Economists may argue that the policy is too costly because the cost per day in a hospital is more expensive than the cost per day at home or in a residential home; yet the most expensive case is not the one that is treated but the one that never goes home.

There are times of rising and times of falling. The seeds of the present come from trees of the past. Anyone who has stayed with me to the end will recognise that if they returned to my beginning and changed the words 'the chronic sick' to 'aged' in the summary of Marjory Warren's (1946) paper, they would find a hypothesis that fits my conclusions. Her hypothesis, formulated in 1946, was based on her work which showed that the chronic sick could be treated. Mine, reflecting my observations and those of many others, is based on my conclusion that British geriatric medicine has shown that it is possible to reduce dependency in the aged by a positive approach to their management.

REFERENCES

Adams, G. F. (1961). Dr. Marjory W. Warren, CBE — 1897–1960. *Gerontol. Clin.*, **3**, 1

Arnold, J. and Exton-Smith, A. N. (1962). The Geriatric Department and the community: value of hospital treatment in the aged. *Lancet*, **ii**, 551

Bagnall, W. E., Datta, S., Knox, J. and Horrocks, P. (1977). Geriatric medicine in Hull: a comprehensive service. *Br. Med. J.*, **2**, 102

Bettman, O. L. (1956). *Pictorial History of Medicine*. Charles C. Thomas, Springfield, Ill.

Brocklehurst, J. C. and Andrews, K. (1985). Geriatric medicine — the style of practice. *Age and Ageing*, **14**, 1

Cross, V. H. (1977). Geriatric medicine — death and rebirth. *Br. Med. J.*, **2**, 816

Das Gupta, P. K. (1980). Developing an active geriatric medical service in Scunthorpe. *Publ. Hlth Lond.*, **94**, 155

Department of Health and Social Security (1981). *Report of a Study on the Respective Roles of the General Acute and Geriatric Sectors in the Care of the Elderly Hospital Patient*. HMSO, London

Exton-Smith, A. N. and Millard, P. H. (1973). To *Hospital Conference* organised by Department of Health and Social Security and British Geriatrics Society, 23 November 1973

Feldstein, M. S. (1963). Operational research and efficiency in the Health Service. *Lancet*, **1**, 491

Graham, J. M. (1983). Experimental nursing homes for elderly people in the National Health Service. *Age and Ageing*, **12**, 273

Grimley-Evans, J. (1983). Integration of geriatric with general medical services in Newcastle. *Lancet*, **ii**, 1430

Grimley-Evans, J. and Graham, J. M. (1984). Medical care of the elderly: Five years on. *J. Roy. Coll. Phys.*, **18**, 18

Hodkinson, H. M. and Jeffreys, P. M. (1972). Making hospital geriatrics work. *Br. Med. J.*, **4**, 536

Howell, T. H. (1974). Origins of the British Geriatrics Society. *Age and Ageing*, **3**, 69

I Ching (1951). *Book of Changes*. Routledge and Kegan Paul paperback edition, London, 1984

Irvine, R. R. (1984). Geriatric medicine and general internal medicine. *J. Roy. Coll. Phys.*, **18**, 21

Kaplan, J. (1983). Planning the future of institutional care: the true costs. *Gerontologist*, **4**, 411

Kayser-Jones, J. S. (1981). *Old, Alone and Neglected: Care of the Aged in Scotland and the United States*, p. 151. University of California Press, London

Leonard, C. J. (1976). Can geriatrics survive? *Br. Med. J.*, **1**, 1335

Means, R. and Smith, R. (1983). From public assistance institutions to 'Sunshine Hotels'; changing State perceptions about residential care for elderly people 1939–48. *Ageing and Society*, **3**, 157

Millard, P. H. (1978). To rehabilitate or to vegetate? *Nursing Mirror*, **146**, 14

Millard, P. H. (1984). Options in the NHS. *Hlth Soc. Serv. J.*, **94**, 852

Nascher, I. L. (1909). *Geriatrics: The Diseases of Old Age and Their Treatment*, p. 517. Blakiston, Philadelphia

O'Brien, T. D., Joshi, D. M. and Warren, E. W. (1973). No apology for geriatrics. *Br. Med. J.*, **4**, 277

Pfeiffer, E. (1985). Some basic principles of working with older patients. *J. Am. Geriat. Soc.*, **33**, 44

Rosen, G. (1967). *The Hospital. Historical Sociology of a Community Institution*. Collier Macmillan, London

Royal College of Physicians (London) (1977). Medical care of the elderly. Report of the Working Party of the Royal College of Physicians, London. *Lancet*, **1**, 1092

Smith, J. (1752). *Portrait of Old Age*, 3rd edn. Withers, London

Somerville Hastings (1951). Old people. *Lancet*, **ii**, 879

Stearns, P. N. (1977). *Old Age in European Society: The Case of France*. Croom Helm, London

Thom, R. (1975). *Structural Stability and Morphogenesis. An Outline of a General Theory of Models*. Benjamin, Reading, Mass.

Thompson, D. (1983). Workhouse to nursing homes: residential care of elderly people in England since 1840. *Ageing and Society*, **3**, 43

Warren, M. R. (1943). Care of the chronic sick: a case for treating chronic sick in blocks in a general hospital. *Br. Med. J.*, **ii**, 822

Warren, M: W. (1946). Care of the chronic aged sick. *Lancet*, **i**, 841

Williamson, J. (1979). Notes on the historical development of geriatric medicine as a specialty. *Age and Ageing*, **8**, 144

Wilson, L. A. (1972). Geriatrics at the crossroads. *Gerontol. Clin.*, **14**, 193

12

The Elderly and High Technology Therapies

Bryan Jennett

INTRODUCTION

The attitudes to high technology medicine of advocates for the elderly are sometimes confused and conflicting. Believing that one reason for the inadequate provision of long-term care for the elderly is overprovision of high technology medicine, some urge a transfer of resources from the acute sector hospitals. The assumption that high technology is mostly used for younger patients overlooks the appropriate need that many elderly patients have for acute medical care. A policy that led to stricter rationing of high technology could disadvantage the elderly by limiting their access to necessary treatment, because when there is rationing, advanced age is a readily applied and widely accepted criterion for exclusion (Jennett, 1987a).

Some advocates urge that there is already unjustified discrimination against the elderly when it comes to choosing patients for such technologies as intensive care or major surgery or dialysis (Avorn, 1984). They fear that increasing insistence on cost–benefit analysis when deciding about the provision of care at both the macro- and micro-allocation levels may disadvantage the elderly. This is because of the emphasis in terms of benefit on the expected duration of survival after treatment as well as on the limited social contribution that older rescued patients can make compared with breadwinners or parents of young children. But the cost side of the equation also poses a problem because of the need, when calculating the cost of securing the benefit of a successful outcome, to include expenditure on all the patients whose treatment proved unsuccessful. Fewer elderly patients have good outcomes than do younger patients treated with the same technology, provided that patients in both series have illness of the same severity.

However, high technology doctors are sometimes accused of overtreating elderly patients in that they seem to take insufficient notice of the limited prospects of success in such patients (Leaf, 1977). Critical illness in the elderly is often terminal illness, and high technology interventions may simply prolong the process of dying. Others whose condition is not yet terminal suffer from chronic disease that is far advanced; interventions may then serve only to extend survival when the quality of life has already become unacceptable to the patient. Whenever treatment for the elderly is unsuccessful or is unkind, it may be deemed to have been inappropriate both on humanitarian and on economic grounds. Policies that purport to benefit the elderly by improving their access to high technology therapies should also consider how to ensure that such inappropriate use is minimised.

High technology therapy for the elderly therefore poses complex problems for decision-makers. Most of these are about the basis of selection, either for active intervention or for limited treatment. The most important influence on this decision should be reliable data about the probability that the treatment in question will benefit a particular patient. There are biological factors that reduce the likelihood of a medically successful outcome as age advances. Whether medical success is regarded as beneficial to the patient is a different but equally important consideration. It may be possible to rescue a patient from impending death, but whether that is a desirable objective is another matter. The elderly patient, his family and his doctors may each have different views about this. Age certainly influences how patients regard the risks and discomforts of therapy and also their perception of disability — how much they are prepared to put up with or what hazards they are willing to face in order to extend life or to reduce disability.

Advocates for the elderly who maintain that age should never be a factor in making decisions about treatment do not serve the best interests of those whom they are claiming to protect. It can be positively disadvantageous for the elderly to be exposed to the rigours of some therapies that might be appropriate for patients half their age. Neither is it sensible to prescribe an upper age limit on access to therapy without linking this to the severity of illness and other aspects of physiological fitness, as well as to the patient's preferences and social situation. The aim should be to give age its appropriate place when making decisions about the initiation and continuation of rescue therapy that involves high technology.

USE OF HIGH TECHNOLOGY BY THE ELDERLY

About 14 per cent of the population in the United Kingdom is over 65 years of age, but this age group is disproportionately represented in admissions to intensive care units (ICUs) and to surgical wards (Table 12.1). In six general

Table 12.1 Percentage of elderly patients in ICU admissions. Source: Jennett (1985)

		Age (years)				
	n	*> 60*	*> 65*	*> 70*	*> 75*	*References*
General ICUs						
UK	3040		31			Table 12.2
US	674	44		22		Knaus *et al.* (1982)
France	586	31		15		Knaus *et al.* (1982)
Coronary care						
Glasgow (confirmed infarct)	503	59	52	21		Williams *et al.* (1976)
Florence						
all cases	2056	52			20	Marchionni *et al.* (1983)
Rt heart catheter	448	59		30		Marchionni *et al.* (1981)
Non-traumatic coma (US/UK)	310	54				Bates *et al.* (1977)
Cardiopulmonary resuscitation (Nuremberg)	335	71				Fusgen and Summa (1978)

ICUs in Britain the average proportion of over 65 years was 31 per cent, with a range of 24–46 per cent (Table 12.2). In one large ICU in the United

Table 12.2 Elderly in UK ICUs. Source: Personal communications

Hospital	*n*	Proportion of admissions (%) *> 65 years*	Mortality (%)	
			< 65 years	*> 65 years*
Barts	432	24	27	23
Bristol	693	25	22	24
Newcastle	606	38	14	17
Glasgow	215	29	20	39
Whipps Cross	401	46	10	26
Middlesex	693	26	5	28

States 44 per cent of patients were over 65 years of age, when only 17 per cent of its catchment population were in this age group; 21 per cent of admissions were over 75 years old, yet this group made up only 5 per cent of the population. In several countries the elderly now account for more than half the admissions to coronary care units, and almost three-quarters of the patients who had cardiopulmonary resuscitation in one German intensive care unit were over the age of 60.

According to a survey in England and Wales (Seymour, 1985), 25 per cent of all surgical admissions are now over 65 years of age and 10 per cent are over 75. In ophthalmological and urological wards 50 per cent are elderly; some series of open heart operations now show 20 per cent over 65 and 10 per cent over 70 years. The age-specific admission rate of over-85-year-olds to surgical wards in general is double that in the age group 45–64, and in trauma and orthopaedic wards it doubles with each decade after 65.

Excluding those to psychiatric wards, 43 per cent of all admissions to hospital over 65 years in England and Wales are to surgical wards; for over-75s the proportion is 38 per cent. Indeed, surgeons now admit as many patients over 75 as do general physicians and geriatricians combined. In the United States a third of all hospital admissions over 65 years of age have an operation (for surgical admissions it is likely to be higher than this, presuming that not all of them have surgery).

The difficulty of defining 'the elderly' is illustrated by Table 12.1. With 65 years a common retiring age and also the age at which patients become eligible for care in geriatric units in the United Kingdom and qualifying for Medicare in the United States, it seems a sensible watershed. However, some reports classify patients by decades, while others focus on patients over 75. It is necessary, therefore, to check that similar age categories are being considered when comparing series.

As older patients more often become ill, it might not seem surprising that they figure disproportionately in series of patients having certain therapeutic interventions. The figures from Britain do not suggest that rationing policies are preventing the access of elderly patients to these technologies. A comparative study of the United States and the United Kingdom (Aaron and Schwartz, 1984) found no evidence of discrimination in Britain against the elderly who required radiotherapy for cancer, while finding that elderly patients with renal failure in the United Kingdom are much less often treated by dialysis than they are in the United States. This difference was attributed to the fact that cancer is perceived as a dread disease that evokes a reflex reaction to active treatment, even though the benefits expected are very limited. With critical illness of the kind that is now considered to require intensive care, it is equally difficult to resist the urge to treat, even though the patient is old and the outlook poor. Certainly, the prospects of a reasonable period of good-quality survival for well-selected elderly patients treated by dialysis can be much better than for many of the older patients who are admitted to intensive care units or who are treated by major surgery or radiotherapy for cancer.

INFLUENCE OF AGE ON OUTCOME

There are two main biological reasons why elderly patients as a group have less likelihood of surviving after critical illness or major surgery; and if they do survive, of making a good recovery. One is that the frequency of multiple pathology is greater than in younger patients, although this does not apply to all elderly patients. Much more important is that the functional reserve capacity of many organs declines linearly from the age of 30, after which mortality doubles every eight years (Fries, 1980). The consequence of this is that disorders of physiological function consequent on accident or illness that would probably be withstood by a younger person can soon become irreversible in the elderly, owing to the inadequate reserve of the organ(s) affected. However, the physiological capacity of healthy older people varies over a wide range. Although on *average* maximum performance declines at 1 per cent a year between 30 and 70 years of age, there are occasional 70-year-olds able to run a marathon in less than four hours. As a guide to the capacity of an individual to recover from critical illness or to withstand major surgery, chronological age alone is unreliable. Some estimate is needed of physiological function and also of the extent of pathology, both in the organ that is to be treated and in other systems. Indeed, a major factor influencing the outcome of surgery in the elderly is the location and extent of pre-operative medical disease.

INTENSIVE CARE

Some general ICUs report similar mortality rates for patients who are over or under 65 years, while in other units older patients have a higher mortality (Table 12.2). The explanation of this surprising finding is likely to lie in differing admission policies. Those units with equally good outcomes in older patients have presumably set criteria for excluding older patients with features likely to be associated with complications and a poor outcome. To what extent such policies may have denied potential benefit to some of the older patients so excluded must be a matter of conjecture. Such figures do not, however, permit of the conclusion that advancing age does not influence outcome; instead they indicate that in carefully selected elderly patients intensive care can give good results.

When patients whose severity of illness is similar are compared then age is found to be a powerful predictor of outcome. For example, in patients in coma after severe head injury, mortality increases with age (Figure 12.1). Indeed the odds on death after severe head injury increase by 3.6 per cent for each year over 35 and decrease at a similar rate below this, and there is no watershed at 50, 60 or 70 years of age (Teasdale *et al.*, 1982). When patients are divided into three degrees of severity (but all of them severely injured), the slope of the line linking age and death rate is the same but the setting is different; a younger patient is more likely to survive a more severe injury than an older patient (Figure 12.2).

The effect of age on outcome is well seen in one large American series which also showed that mortality after leaving the ICU/CCU rose with age (Table 12.3). Two non-medical American authors drew attention to the fact

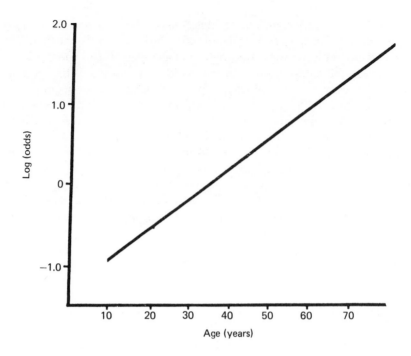

Figure 12.1 Patients with severe head injury (more than 6 hours in coma). log (odds) on death increase with age. Source: Teasdale *et al.* (1982)

that 20 per cent of the annual Medicare budget was spent on the 5 per cent patients who died in that year — many of them deaths in ICUs of patients over 65 years who now comprise the largest age group among the terminally ill (Bayer *et al.*, 1983). They commented that while it would be wrong to deny care to the dying because there would be no economic return, it would be unjust to patients who could benefit if priority were given to the terminally ill.

It is not surprising that more than half the patients in coronary care units (CCUs) are over 65 years, because heart disease is the commonest cause of death in this age group. Many of these deaths are premature and potentially preventable, and elderly patients may stand to benefit more than younger patients from admission to a CCU. One reason is that heart block and cardiac arrhythmias occur twice as frequently over the age of 70 years. The other is that older patients are particularly vulnerable to the consequences of abrupt reduction in cardiac output, especially its effect on the brain. If such crises are promptly detected and dealt with, there is a better chance of survival and the avoidance of disability in survivors.

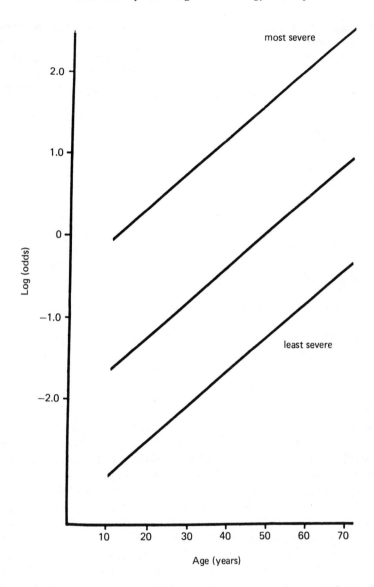

Figure 12.2   log (odds) on death after severe head injury. Lines are parallel but set at different levels according to degree of severity of brain damage. Source: Teasdale *et al.* (1982)

Table 12.3 MGH — 2693 admissions to Medical ICU + CCU — (1977–79) (derived from Campion *et al.*, 1981)

	Age (years)			
	55–64	*65–74*	*> 75*	*> 65*
Percentage of admissions in each age group	24	23	21	44
Percentage having major interventions of each age group	22	26	32	
Cumulative mortality (%)				
in ICU/CCU	5	8	22	9
in hospital	8	14	33	15
within 1 year	10	16	43	38
Mortality in myocardial infarct cases (%)				
in hospital	9	21	29	–
1 year	15	30	42	–

Note: MGH = Massachusetts General Hospital

SURGERY

As with intensive care, there are some surgical series that show mortality rates for older patients that differ little from those of younger patients (Table 12.4). As with good results from intensive care in the elderly, these figures doubtless reflect a rigorous selection policy. By contrast, a review of the post-operative mortality in 17 000 general surgical cases in Finland showed that only 20 per cent of patients were over 70 years but that 91 per cent of the deaths were in these elderly patients (Palmberg and Hirsjarvi, 1979). The overall mortality was 9 per cent in 590 elderly patients, but after emergency operations it was 37 per cent, compared with 8 per cent for elective procedures. The mortality in older patients with dementia was 45 per cent, with diabetes 26 per cent and with cardiac disease 17 per cent. Death was seldom due to surgical complications, and less than 10 per cent died directly from their primary disease. The commonest causes of death were pulmonary embolism and cardiac complications during or after operation.

A review of 505 surgical admissions over 65 years in Scotland showed that only half had an operation (Table 12.5). There were as many deaths among those who did not come to surgery as among those who did. Mortality from emergency operations was more than four times higher than for elective procedures. Mortality for all admissions (with or without surgery) was more

Table 12.4 Cardiac surgery in elderly patients
  (a) Open heart surgery (in Glasgow) (source: D. Wheatley, personal communication)

	n	*Percentage of procedures* > 65 years	*Operative mortality (%)* < 65 years	> 65 years
CABG	447	10	4.2	4.4
Valve replacement	187	14	8.1	3.7
Both	40	25	7.5	0
Total	674	12	5.6	3.7

(b) Mortality in published series

	n	*Age* (years)	%	*Reference*
Valve replacement	135	> 70	8	Arom *et al.* (1984)
Aortic valve	62	> 70	8	Glock *et al.* (1984)
Cardiac surgery	25	> 80	4	Rich *et al.* (1985)

Table 12.5 Mortality (%) of elderly surgical patients (in parentheses, excluding 'non-viable'). Derived from Seymour and Pringle (1982)

n =	*All admissions* 505	*After operation* 205	*No operation* 148	*Minor procedures* 97
All > 65 years	15 (3)	12 (6)	24 (2)	6 (0)
65–74 years	10 (1)	–		
> 75 years	21 (7)	–		
Elective operation	–	7 (1)		
Emergency operation	–	26 (7)		

than twice as high for over-75-year-olds as for those aged 65–74. This review emphasised that many patients were already moribund on admission; these non-viable patients accounted for half the operative deaths and almost all the deaths in patients who did not have surgery. More than two-thirds of these non-viable patients had inoperable malignancies, some of whom were nonetheless submitted to surgery.

All series show that emergency surgery has a higher mortality, and there is evidence also that the proportion of operations that are emergencies increases with age (30 per cent for 45–64-year-olds, 40 per cent age 65–74 and 50 per cent over 75 years) (Seymour and Pringle, 1983). Elderly patients presenting as emergencies often have advanced disease, and may be in a poor state of general health, nutrition and hydration. There is also less time to assess coexisting medical conditions before operation, while procedures undertaken out of normal working hours often involve less experienced surgeons and anaesthetists. It seems likely that if there were guidelines about withholding emergency surgery from non-viable patients and delaying the operation in some others, there might be less unsuccessful surgery performed on elderly patients who present as emergencies.

DECISIONS ABOUT HIGH TECHNOLOGY TREATMENT

Certain principles of medical ethics proposed as action guides by Beauchamp and Childress (1983) are useful in making these decisions. These are best expressed as questions:

- *Beneficence*   What is the probability that life of reasonable quality and duration will be restored by treatment? What is the probability of improving the outcome compared with that expected if the intervention is withheld?
- *Non-maleficence*   How much hazard, distress and indignity are likely to be associated with the proposed intervention? What are the risks of early mortality or complications from surgery, and what are the chances that intensive care may result either in incomplete recovery or in prolonging life that is already of poor quality.
- *Patient autonomy*   When informed of the balance of probabilities, what is the patient's preference?

When older patients are given an opportunity to express their own views about technologies such as intensive care, surgery, cardiopulmonary resuscitation or dialysis, it becomes clear that their attitudes and their goals are often different from those of their doctors. Older patients are often willing to accept higher risks of early post-operative death than are their surgeons. But they are often less willing to have resuscitation or prolonged intensive care or dialysis than their doctors are to provide it. Elderly people often harbour fears that they may be kept alive when they would prefer to have been allowed to die, and they are also concerned that when that time comes, they may themselves no longer be competent to make their wishes known — in particular, to withhold consent. This has led in America to the living will or right-to-die movements. In the absence of such formal declaration, relatives may claim to know what the wishes of the patient would have been; but this should be assessed with care, because there may be a conflict of interests between the elderly patient and his family.

Although formal consent is traditionally always sought before surgical procedures are undertaken, this is not usual before embarking on intensive care, dialysis or cardiopulmonary resuscitation (Jennett, 1984). Indeed, intensive care is often the result of a step-wise process that begins with post-operative care. Some surgeons insist that once a decision has been made to operate on an elderly patient, then no effort should be spared to provide post-operative intensive care without limit, even if major complications develop (Reiss, 1980). Such surgeons are victims of the cycle of commitment which I have illustrated by this example from a regional neurosurgical unit (Jennett, 1986).

> On the telephone he sounded better than he now is and he was thought to be only 65 years of age. On admission he is found to be 75 years old, with fixed dilated pupils and flaccid limbs. All known evidence predicts that he cannot recover. But it is argued that as he has come 30 miles by ambulance the least that can be done is a CT scan. This shows a large intracranial haematoma. Even so, the evidence is that recovery is not possible even with prompt surgery, given his clinical state and age. But having discovered a surgical lesion the argument again runs that it is difficult to let it be. The trainee surgeon wonders what his chief (or the coroner) will say if he leaves it untreated. So surgery is performed but at the end of the operation the patient will not breathe on his own. Is the decision to let him die in the operating room or the recovery room? No, that is not good for the surgical statistics, for the anaesthetic audit or for the morale of the nurses in the operating room. So the patient goes to the ICU on a ventilator. Next day he can breathe a little on his own but otherwise is no better. Because he is not brain dead there may be no one prepared to make the overdue decision to withdraw the ventilator and he may linger for several days before death comes.

Elderly patients are more likely to develop complications after surgery or to fail to recover rapidly after resuscitation or after intensive care has been instituted. There should, therefore, be an undertaking before embarking on such therapies in old people that a prolonged and futile period of continued treatment will not be allowed to happen by default. If there were a clear policy for withdrawing or scaling down treatment once it had become clear that there could not be a successful outcome, there might be less reluctance to offer elderly patients the opportunity to benefit from such technologies (Jennett, 1987b).

It is significant that, although the rate of admission for emergency surgery rises steadily with increasing age, admissions for elective surgery fall off after 65 years in Britain, which suggests a reluctance to perform elective surgery in patients of this age. Evidence for this also comes from the difference between the UK and the US rates for some common elective procedures — a difference that becomes more marked after the age of 65 years. There may, therefore, be an unmet need in this age group because

surgeons are withholding treatment from some older patients who could
benefit. This may be because risks are considered to be higher than they
really are, or that the surgeons underestimate the expectations of life. For fit
men of 75 years of age this is 6 years and for women 9 years, in Britain. A
study of surgical patients in Denmark showed 46 per cent of 70-year-olds
alive ten years after operation; for those with no coexisting medical
condition the ten-year survival was 66 per cent (Anderson and Ostberg,
1972a,b). These rates are much better than those that are common after
major surgery for cancer in patients aged 46–64 years — yet such treatment
is rarely withheld.

CONCLUSION

What matters is that age be given its appropriate place when making
decisions about the initiation and continuation of rescue therapy (Jennett,
1985). Whether or not treatment is appropriate depends on whether there is
a reasonable chance of restoring life of quality for long enough to be worth
the burden of treatment to the patient, to the family and to society. It also
depends on a reasonable certainty that intervention will not do more harm
than good — a value judgement about the balance of burdens and benefits
(Jennett, 1986). It should also be ensured that what is done is what the
patient wishes or would have wanted were he or she able to express a
preference. Doctors should also be satisfied that they are neither denying
treatment nor insisting on it for the benefit of themselves rather than of the
patient. No elderly patient should be denied access to a procedure in order
to preserve the statistics of success in a series to be reported, because this
may deprive an old person of a reasonable chance of relief. But neither
should an elderly patient be treated simply to avoid the trouble of defending
a charge of inadequate care when to intervene would be against that
patient's best interest.

A useful safeguard against inappropriate treatment is for institutions (or
individual services within them) to evolve written guidelines about recommended practice for rescue therapy at all ages. This prior consensus should
be derived from the best available data about prognosis. It is dishonest to
hide behind a cloak of supposed ignorance and pretend not to know who will
and who will not respond to therapy. For many situations good data are
available about the expected outcome at different ages. Decisions should be
based on data — not on slogans, on impulses or on cowardice.

REFERENCES

Aaron, H. J. and Schwartz, W. B. (1984). *The Painful Prescription: Rationing
Hospital Care*. The Brookings Institutions, Washington D.C.

Anderson, B. and Ostberg, J. (1972a). Survival rates in surgery of the aged. Assessment of long-term prognosis according to coexisting disease. *Gerontol. Clin.*, **14**, 354

Anderson, B. and Ostberg, J. (1972b). Long-term prognosis in geriatric surgery: 2–17 year follow-up of 7922 patients. *J. Am. Geriat. Soc.*, **20**, 255

Arom, K. V., Nicoloff, D. M., Lindsay, W. G., Northrup, W. F. and Kertsen, T. E. (1984). Should valve replacement and related procedures be performed in elderly patients. *Ann. Thorac. Surg.*, **39**, 466

Avorn, J. (1984). Benefit and cost analysis in geriatric care: turning age discrimination into health policy. *New Engl. J. Med.*, **310**, 1294

Bates, D., Caronna, J. J., Cartlidge, N. E. F., Knill-Jones, R. P., Levy, D. E., Shaw, D. A. and Plum, F. (1977). A prospective study of non-traumatic coma: methods and results in 310 patients. *Ann. Neurol.*, **2**, 215

Bayer, R., Callahan, D., Fletcher, J., Hodgson, T., Jennings, B., Monsees, D., Sieverts, S. and Veatch, R. (1983). The care of the terminally ill: morality and economics. *New Engl. J. Med.*, **309**, 1490

Beauchamp, T. L. and Childress, J. F. (1983). *Principles of Biomedical Ethics*, 2nd edn. Oxford University Press, New York

Campion, E. W., Mulley, A. G., Goldstein, R. L., Barnett, G. O. and Thibault, G. E. (1981). Medical intensive care for the elderly: a study of current use, costs and outcomes. *J. Am. Med. Ass.*, **246**, 2052

Fries, J. F. (1980). Aging, natural death, and the compression of morbidity. *New Engl. J. Med.*, **303**, 130

Fusgen, I. and Summa, J.-D. (1978). How much sense is there in an attempt to resuscitate an aged person? *Gerontology*, **24**, 37

Glock, T., Pecoul, R., Cerene, A., Laguerre, J. and Pull, P. (1984). Aortic valve replacement in elderly patients. *J. Cardiovasc. Surg.*, **25**, 205

Jennett, B. (1984). Inappropriate use of intensive care. *Br. Med. J.*, **289**, 1709

Jennett, B. (1985). Intensive care for the elderly. *Int. J. Tech. Assess. Hlth Care*, **1**, 7

Jennett, B. (1986). *High Technology Medicine — Benefits and Burdens*, 2nd edn. Oxford University Press, Oxford

Jennett, B. (1987a). High technology medicine and the elderly. *Int. J. Tech. Assess. Hlth Care* (in press)

Jennett, B. (1987b). Decisions to limit treatment. *Lancet*, **2**, 787

Knaus, W. W., Draper, E. A., Wagner, D. P., Zimmerman, J. E., Birnbaum, M. L., Cullen, D. J., Kohles, M. K., Shin, B. and Snyder, J. V. (1982). Evaluating outcome from intensive care: a preliminary multihospital comparison. *Crit. Care Med.*, **10**, 491

Knaus, W. A., Le Gall, J. R., Wagner, D. P., Draper, E. A., Loirat, P., Campos, R. A., Cullen, D. J., Kohles, M. K., Glaser, P., Granthil, C., Mercier, P., Nicolas, F., Nikki, P., Shim, B., Snyder, J. V., Wattel, J. V. and Zimmerman, J. E. (1982). A comparison of intensive care in the USA and France. *Lancet*, **2**, 642

Leaf, A. (1977). Medicine and the aged. *New Engl. J. Med.*, **297**, 887

Marchionni, N., Pini, R., Vanucci, A., Calamandrei, M., Conti, A., Di Bari, M., Greppi, B. and Antonini, F. M. (1981). Intensive care for the elderly with acute myocardial infarction. *J. Clin. Exp. Gerontol.*, **3**, 47

Marchionni, N., Pini, R., Vanucci, A., Greppi, B., Ferrucci, L., Conti, A., Di Bari, M., Calamandrei, M., De Alfieri, W., and Moschi, G. (1983). Acute myocardial infarction in the elderly: a review of 2056 cases. *J. Clin. Exp. Gerontol.*, **5**, 265

Palmberg, S. and Hirsjarvi, E. (1979). Mortality in geriatric surgery. *Gerontology*, **25**, 103

Reiss, R. (1980). Moral and ethical issues in geriatric surgery. *J. Med. Ethics*, **6**, 7

Rich, M. W., Sandza, J. G., Kleiger, R. E. and Connors, J. P. (1985). Cardiac operations in patients over 80 years of age. *J. Thorac. Cardiovasc. Surg.*, **90**, 56

Seymour, G. (1985). *Medical Assessment of the Elderly Surgical Patient*. Croom Helm, London

Seymour, G. and Pringle, R. (1982). A new method of auditing surgical mortality rates: application to a group of elderly surgical patients. *Br. Med. J.*, **284**, 1539

Seymour, G. and Pringle, R. (1983). Surgical emergencies in the elderly: can they be prevented. *Hlth Bull. (Edinburgh)*, **41**, 112

Teasdale, G., Skene, A., Spiegelhalter, D. and Murray, L. (1982). Age, severity and outcome of head injury. In Grossman, R. G. and Gildenberg, P. L. (Eds.), *Head Injury: Basic and Clinical Aspects*. Raven Press, New York

Williams, B. O., Begg, T. B. and McGuinness, J. B. (1976). The elderly in a coronary unit. *Br. Med. J.*, **2**, 451

13

The Community Care Approach: An Innovation in Home Care by Social Services Departments

David Challis and Bleddyn Davies

INTRODUCTION

In the United Kingdom long-term care in the community is emerging as a reality for a number of client groups. These include the chronically and episodically mentally ill, the mentally handicapped, the severely physically handicapped and the dependent elderly. Government policies which are concerned to reduce the reliance upon institutional solutions for the care of these individuals have combined with demographic pressure due to increasing numbers of very elderly people and constrained budgets to focus our attention upon these long-term care groups. However, the development of successful policies for effective care in the community is hampered by the lack of appropriate service models and structures to respond to need (Audit Commission, 1986). Indeed, it is likely that both the Health Service and social services are, on the whole, better geared to provide care for shorter episodes or more acute forms of intervention in the community or to provide community support to the less dependent.

The frail elderly requiring long-term care in their own homes have a great variety of needs stemming from the degree and type of mental impairment suffered, the extent of their physical disability, the amount of family and neighbourly support available, and the time, duration and preference for types of care. This wide variety of needs does not correspond to the relatively inflexible and limited range of services available. The help provided is thus often only a partial solution to people's needs and does not necessarily respond to their preferences. Furthermore, these services are organisationally highly fragmented, coming from a wide range of sources both formal and informal, including the Social Services Department, the National Health Service, family, friends and neighbours. As a consequence, the picture of resource provision for the frail elderly is all too often that of a series of piecemeal contributions from a range of different services, with no one having an unambiguous responsibility for taking a broader view of need beyond their particular remit. Assessments and care plans tend, therefore, to be 'service-oriented' rather than 'client-centred', piecemeal and not holistic, defining needs in terms of available services of care rather than individual problems. Even where appropriate assessments and care plans are effected, these are rarely closely monitored and therefore fail to keep pace with changes in the health and dependency of the elderly person.

The lack of any one person clearly responsible for cementing together these fragmented services into a coherent package is a significant factor militating against their capacity effectively to prevent admission to institutional care. However, an integrated system of care for an individual elderly person has to be consciously created. It will neither happen spontaneously nor arise from simply improving the individual services which are the constituent parts of a care package. In short, a more effective and efficient long-term care system requires both an enhancement of the content of services and also improved case-management (Challis and Davies, 1986; Davies and Challis, 1986).

THE COMMUNITY CARE APPROACH

The Kent Community Care Project was an attempt to provide alternative forms of support in the community to residential and long-stay hospital care for frail elderly people. It was designed to tackle both the problems of the inappropriate content of services, and their fragmentation and lack of co-ordination which inhibit the development of effective long-term care. Social workers were to act as case-managers, and were responsible for the construction and maintenance of individual packages of care unique to each elderly person from the wide range of different and frequently un-coordinated sources of help available. Decisions about the allocation of resources were decentralised to individual field-workers, with defined caseload and expenditure limits to ensure accountability, so that there were greater opportunities for flexible and imaginative solutions to problems.

In order to effect these desired changes from common practice in care of the elderly (Stevenson and Parsloe, 1978; Goldberg and Warburton, 1979), the scheme introduced a number of devices.

Focused care The scheme was clearly targeted. Its concern was those people on the margin of entry to institutional care.

Smaller caseloads and more experienced staff Although it is common for those working with the elderly to have large caseloads, the norms for work in the scheme were not dissimilar to those working with vulnerable children, about 25–30 cases. This was designed to facilitate careful and continuing assessment and monitoring of needs, effective liaison with other agencies, closer and regular contact with the elderly person and their network, and to provide the opportunity to develop community resources such as neighbourly help.

Decentralised budgets   The social workers had control of a decentralised budget to enable them to extend the range of possible solutions for client problems. All the expenditure of existing social services such as home help or meals-on-wheels was notionally charged to the budget as well as actual additional expenditure upon new services or community resources. Hence, an awareness of the unit costs of different services and alternative ways of meeting need was brought into field workers' decisions. In order to balance this greater autonomy in the allocation of resources with the requirements of an accountable agency, expenditure upon individual cases was limited to two-thirds of the cost of a place in a residential home, with expenditure above that limit requiring management sanction. This 'accountability ceiling' placed the freedom of frontline staff within clearly defined parameters.

Closer links with health care   Although the budget spanned the services of only one agency, it was hoped that through the 'give and take' of service provision more effective local collaboration would develop, particularly with the geriatric service and community nursing. Wherever possible, therefore, the area covered by the scheme was coterminous with that of relevant sectors of the Health Service.

Systematic recording   In order further to enhance accountability and promote good practice, systematic records were developed which dealt with information about assessment, regular case reviews and weekly costs for each case. These records could provide feedback to individual workers about their caseload management, and at a more aggregated level assist in management, supervision and strategic planning (Challis and Chesterman, 1985, 1986, 1987).

This, then, is the Community Care Scheme model. A number of Social Services Departments have developed services based upon all or most of these characteristics, and several of these are currently being monitored. In Gateshead a small joint health and social care pilot project is also being undertaken.

THE SCHEME AND CARE OF THE ELDERLY

It was particularly noticeable that the greater flexibility of response afforded to social workers and the provision of a decentralised budget provided an environment where *assessment of need* could be more effective. The approach was 'problem-oriented' rather than the assessment of elderly people in relation to their eligibility for a standard service. The identification of needs was separated from consideration of the means of tackling them, the incentive to undertake coherent assessment coming from the capacity to respond in different ways to individual needs. The continuing responsibility for cases, monitoring closely the care of elderly people, meant that frequently further needs which were not initially apparent would be uncovered, and responses were required for these, often in ways that are not usually possible with the available range of services. This might, for example, mean finding ways of helping people to adjust to significant life changes.

The use of existing resources of the Social Services Department, although often in different ways and at different times, proved to be an important part of care for the majority of cases. The additional budget was used in a variety of ways, such as the purchase of aids and materials not usually available. However, the most frequent solution which it provided was the recruitment of local people as helpers, to assist elderly people in a variety of ways, carefully interwoven with the contribution of established services. The tasks which helpers have undertaken have ranged from immediately practical help with tasks of daily living to the social and therapeutic, such as accompanying a phobic old lady on walks of gradually increasing length, reactivating old interests and abilities or more simple companionship. When helpers were introduced to clients, they were given a 'contract' making explicit the agreed tasks and objectives of care, which clarified the expectations of the agency in providing a fee and reduced uncertainty. Care was taken to try and 'match' elderly persons and helpers, to attempt to ensure that both relational and instrumental needs are met. Helpers have a wide range of backgrounds, from those with previous caring experience, either professionally, such as retired nurses or home helps, or informally within their own families to those with space in their lives which they wished to fill with worth-while activity, such as young housewives or the recently bereaved.

Among other responses was the development of small day-care groups of four or five elderly people in a helper's home to undertake social and rehabilitative activities. This proved particularly useful for people unsuited to more traditional forms of day care. Short-term care in helpers' homes was also arranged following periods of illness or hospitalisation.

The capacity of the social worker as case-manager to respond more effectively could also be seen in the response made to problems which often prove very difficult to manage within the usual range of services. One example is the *risk of falling* for elderly people living alone. Not uncommonly, the fear of this event and the likely damage from the subsequent 'long lie' (Hall, 1982) may be sufficient for the elderly person to relinquish independent living, as a response both to his or her own anxiety and to that of others. However, where their preference to remain at home was strong, it seemed that a well-coordinated plan of regular visiting and, where appropriate, an alarm system could often be sufficient to alleviate the anxiety of the elderly person and other carers and enable him or her to remain at home.

Elderly people suffering from *minor psychiatric disorders* such as depression and anxiety frequently receive inappropriate services compared with otherwise similarly needy people, and the condition is frequently not identified (Foster *et al.*, 1976; Goldberg and Huxley, 1980). In the original scheme it appeared that field workers more frequently identified these problems and took steps to ensure that appropriate treatment was provided. It was observed that, with additional social support and stimulation accompanied by an attention to detail, a positive response was achieved in a considerable proportion of those cases with depressed mood. A small but noteworthy group, 8 per cent of cases, suffered with problems of excessive alcohol intake, often in association with depression and social isolation. About half of these represented long-standing drink problems persisting into old age, and the rest appeared to be of recent onset in response to social stress. Close support and supervision to maintain a level of acceptable or controlled drinking was reasonably successful, in part because sources of supply were known and could be monitored by the case-manager, and attempts were made to mitigate the ill-effects of drink by ensuring the provision of an adequate diet. For the late-onset individuals, considerable efforts were also made to tackle the precipitating stresses such as isolation and loneliness.

Even in the care of the *dementing elderly*, where particularly great care problems are found, there was some degree of success in the establishment and maintenance of care and reduction of risk through a more structured approach (Challis and Davies, 1985, 1986). Often it is difficult to establish, let alone maintain, a package of care for these people. As with other intractable problems, effective care appeared possible as a result of both continuing case management and the capacity to respond in a more individualised way to needs. Thus, help could be made more acceptable and access gained to an individual through a variety of strategies. These included persistence, a response to particular behavioural problems, a willingness initially to provide help where need was recognised by the elderly person rather than where the need appeared greatest, and as much concern about those elements of retained ability as a base for building care as about those areas of increasing deficit.

'Process risk', the not infrequent downward spiral of increasing self-neglect, decline and reduction of coping skills, was tackled by organising care to provide supervision, food, medication and stimulation to arrest nutritional and social decline. 'Event risk' was defined as the loss of coping skills where normal sequential acts of daily living are not completed in their entirety, such as turning on gas-taps and failing to light them, causing a hazard to the elderly person and his or her environment. This was tackled by modifications to the physical environment, such as turning off the gas supply or providing electric kettles which switch off automatically. Other responses to event risk involved identifying regular behaviour patterns which may be repeated and establishing routines with close supervision in order to reduce the risk of wandering. Case management through 'patterning care' involved the construction of a clear and regular pattern of care based initially upon the positive elements retained by the old person despite his or her mental disability. These patterns were, wherever possible, made meaningful within the old person's routine, or dependent upon external cues such as light and dark, night and day. Where there was no such routine, attempts were made to create one (for example, associating particular activities with retiring to bed and perhaps tiring a person at a more appropriate time), so as to provide a more predictable and apparently secure environment.

Support for carers was more readily provided. Existing services, such as a day hospital, day centres or home help, may be only partially effective, perhaps because an elderly person is too sick to attend or the carer does not desire help with domestic tasks. In certain cases what was required was help which fitted with the carer's particular interests, needs or problems, such as regular relief on particular days or evenings, the stimulation of a visitor who could relieve both old person and carer, or, perhaps, help to settle the old person at a specific time. At other times it was necessary to devise with carers realistic boundaries and limits to their involvement, to prevent their being overwhelmed by the day-to-day demands of care or 'polarisation' of the burden onto one family member (Ratna and Davies, 1984).

Discharge from permanent hospital and residential care has proved possible in a few cases, and for others earlier than would otherwise have been the case. This has been possible, as the social workers have been able to plan these activities with sufficient control over resources to respond to the particular needs of individuals, and thereby gain the co-operation of hospital and residential care staff in planned rehabilitation and discharge.

COSTS AND EFFECTIVENESS

A number of the Community Care Schemes are being evaluated, although results are available only for the early projects. The evaluation was undertaken using a quasi-experimental design, comparing similar cases from adjacent areas, both of which were part of the same health and social care system (Davies and Challis, 1981). Interviews were undertaken with elderly people and their carers immediately prior to the scheme intervention and again one year later. Here we present results from the first Kent project and its subsequent 'sister' development in Gateshead.

Effects upon Elderly People and Their Carers

Cases were matched by six factors likely to be predictors of survival in the Community. These were sex, age, living group (household composition), presence of confusion, physical disability and receptivity to help. As a result of this process, 74 matched pairs were identified in the Kent project. The location of the 74 matched pairs over three years is shown in Table 13.1. It

Table 13.1 Location of 74 matched cases over one, two and three years receiving the Community Care Scheme and standard services Kent project

	Year 1		Year 2		Year 3	
	CCS	Std services	CCS	Std services	CCS	Std services
At home	51	25	37	15	26	9
Residential care	9	20	15	25	16	23
Hospital care	3	4	2	2	6	1
Moved away	1	1	1	2	2	2
Died	10	24	19	30	24	39
	74	74	74	74	74	74

can be seen that, after one year, whereas 69 per cent of the Community Care group remained in their own homes, only 34 per cent of the control group did so. This difference was largely to be explained by the different rates of admission to residential care and death. A similar pattern can be observed in favour of the Community Care Scheme over three years. This was unlikely to be an effect of the matching process, since no differences were evident between the groups in terms of functional status, poor memory or other correlates of organic brain disease, and physical frailty was, if anything, greater for the Community Care group. Possible explanations for the differences in survival rate appeared to be the reduced 'relocation effect' (Yawney and Slover, 1973), since fewer Community Care cases entered institutional care and the influence of the extended social support (Berkmann and Syme, 1979) provided by the Community Care Scheme. A third possible explanation is the effect of closer monitoring of the health and social status of frail elderly people, which has been associated with reduced mortality (Luker, 1981; Hendriksen et al., 1984; Vetter et al., 1984).

There were significant improvements in a range of indicators of subjective well-being and quality of care for those receiving Community Care compared with elderly people in receipt of the standard services. Other analyses demonstrated that there was a lower rate of decline in functional status among the Community Care group, which could in part be attributed to close liaison between the Scheme social workers and the geriatric day hospital.

There were also benefits to informal carers. Whereas the Community Care Scheme was significantly more effective in reducing subjective stress among carers, there was no significant different between the Community Care group and the control group in relation to reduction in practical demands upon carers, such as effects upon employment or social life. The explanation for this appeared to be that, in the control group, elderly people with carers were particularly likely to enter institutional care. Entry to institutional care and effective support at home likewise reduce the difficulties in social life or employment. However, a carer who has, through lack of any other option, had to place an elderly relative in institutional care could sometimes experience considerable guilt and distress.

The Costs of Care

The costs of care were compared at a 1977 price base, the year in which the scheme commenced. Costs are shown in Table 13.2 for the Social Services Department, the National Health Service and society as a whole, both as an annual cost and per month survived, since there was a difference in death rate between the two groups. The costs represent the first year's care for a cohort of 74 cases. These average cost figures suggest a clear, if small, cost

Table 13.2   Costs of care over one year (1977 prices) for matched cases receiving the Community Care Scheme and standard services Kent project

	Annual costs (£)		Cost per month (£)[a]	
	CCS	Std services	CCS	Std services
Social Services Department	639	702	52	59
National Health Service	778	708	69	75
Society as a whole[b]	2850	2686	238	265

[a] Cost per month refers to per month survived. It therefore takes account of the shorter survival period of the control group.

[b] Social opportunity costs included health and social care expenditure, the value of private housing, the old person's living expenses and directly observable financial costs borne by carers. The capital costs of hospitals, residential homes and private housing were discounted over a 60 year period at a rate of 7 per cent.

advantage to the Social Services Department from the Community Care Scheme. However, the NHS results suggest little difference in costs due to the two models of care, greater longevity tending to increase costs for the Community Care group. This average cost figure, however, conceals an important difference in its constituent parts. There was a markedly lower utilisation of residential homes and long-stay hospitals for those elderly people receiving the new service, and a correspondingly greater use of domiciliary services, and day hospital and acute hospital facilities. Indeed, in the care of the very dependent, community care appeared to be substituting for long-term hospital care.

Further analysis indicated that there are two groups for whom Community Care is especially cost-effective. The first of these is the extremely dependent person with mental and physical frailty who receives a considerable degree of informal support. This finding would appear to agree with the conclusion of Bergmann *et al.* (1978). The second group is the socially isolated elderly person, with only a moderate degree of dependency, likely to suffer from depression. These are people whose difficulties are frequently undetected in usual circumstances (Foster *et al.*, 1976; Goldberg and Huxley, 1980).

REPLICATION AND DEVELOPMENT

Earlier we noted that our existing structure of services has grown in a somewhat haphazard fashion, often designed for different circumstances from those in which we work today. Most of those services and new developments associated with them have never been subject to rigorous evaluation. Nonetheless, in the current climate it is ever more important '. . . to ensure that care-planning and provision is informed by evidence as well as fashion' (Wattis, 1986). Of course, one evaluation does not constitute sufficient evidence for the adoption of a new approach to care, any more than the sighting of one swallow constitutes proof of the arrival of summer. A number of factors, such as unique features of the local area, staff enthusiasm or the behaviour of other services, could have contributed to the results which we have described. For this reason we have undertaken a replication of the approach in a completely different area, namely North-east England (Challis *et al.*, 1987).

The findings of the Gateshead study confirm those of the original Kent scheme. The greater freedom afforded by specialisation in this area of work and possession of a budget enabled staff to tackle some of the more intractable problems in the community with greater success than is frequently the case. Indeed, the practice developments improved and built upon those of the initial scheme. A follow-up of 90 matched pairs of cases over a twelve-month period indicated that a much higher proportion of people who received the Community Care Scheme remained in their own homes than in the control group (63 per cent, compared with 36 per cent). Only 1 per cent of those who received Community Care were in a residential home after one year, compared with 39 per cent of those who received the usual range of services. The numbers in long-stay hospitals were not dissimilar (Challis *et al.*, 1987). It is clear that these findings are similar to those of the original Kent study, with the exception that there was no significant difference in the death rate.

Analyses of indicators of quality of life and quality of care of elderly people and their carers suggested that those who received the Community Care Scheme were significantly better off than those who received the usual range of services. It was noteworthy that, for those who had survived, of the four possible care options (Community Care and remaining at home; Community Care and entry to institutional care; standard services and remaining at home; standard services and entry to institutional care), three of these options appeared to produce benefits for elderly people and their carers. However, the fourth option — the receipt of standard services and remaining at home — was significantly less effective in meeting needs. This finding is of particular importance, since it is consistent with the recent report of the Audit Commission (1986), which argued that the present organisational arrangements for providing care in the community are simply untenable.

Our comparison of costs in the Gateshead scheme over a one-year period lead to similar conclusions to those which we drew from the Kent scheme — namely, that there is no significant difference between the costs of Community Care and the usual range of services from the point of view of the Social Services Department and the National Health Service. We are engaged in further analyses to identify the characteristics of those cases for whom the scheme proved to be the most and least cost-effective.

CONCLUDING OBSERVATIONS

It would seem that the Community Care approach appeared to provide an environment where what could be described as 'good social work practice' with the elderly can develop. The organisational arrangements provided a means of balancing the greater autonomy of frontline staff with their accountability to the agency. The results suggest a more imaginative, effective and efficient response to need through closer and better-coordinated control of resources by frontline staff. This moves away from a rather blinkered professional outlook to encompass the role of case-manager, responsible for a wide range of resources and their co-ordination, development and control. In so doing, the case-management role bridges the inappropriate split which has existed between social work and social care; that is to say, between the provision of practical help on the one hand, and psychological support on the other. This role could be seen as providing a very clear statement of the nature of the social-work task with elderly people, which has too frequently evaded helpful description in the past (Barclay, 1982). In many instances it proved possible to maintain elderly people at home with improved quality of life for themselves and their carers which traditional services seemed unable to provide. We have also observed that the principles and practice are transferable, since the Gateshead scheme was undertaken in an area with very different socio-economic circumstances.

Our findings, along with early analyses of a replication, suggest that the operation of the scheme in different parts of the United Kingdom has demonstrated that, despite the arbitrary barriers that exist between health and social care, an improved service by one agency can provide benefits for both. The scheme offers a model which would enable Social Services Departments to integrate their services to *all* elderly people. However, given the complex interrelationship between physical, psychiatric, social and emotional problems in the frail elderly, and, indeed, in other long-term-care groups, there is also room for an extension of this approach in terms of joint health and social services activity. This could occur as a part of primary health care services or as part of a community-based geriatric or psychogeriatric service where the key-worker principle is already in place in assessment, care planning and monitoring of patients (Hemsi, 1980).

The prescriptions of the Audit Commission (1986), which argue for a single manager with a single budget to develop community care services for the elderly, has an apparent similarity to the Community Care developments we have outlined. However, the similarity is misleading since the Audit Commission's (1986) proposals seem to be based upon a 'top down' view of organisations. Yet the experience of services in Northern Ireland, with integrated Health and Social Service management, would suggest that there is no necessary concordance between managerial integration and field-professional integration at the client level. The Community Care approach, by contrast, is a 'bottom-up' solution to the fragmentation of care, starting with the co-ordination of care for the individual client or patient. As such it could be one means by which managers of community services for the elderly might deploy their budget, either to individual case managers or to case managers within health and social care teams. Certainly our evidence suggests that the future development of community services could well be considerably enhanced by undertaking an approach which adopted decentralised control of resources and effective case-management in the care of the frail elderly.

REFERENCES

Audit Commission (1986). *Making a Reality of Community Care.* HMSO, London
Barclay, P. (1982). *Social Workers: Their Roles and Tasks.* Bedford Square Press, London
Bergmann, K., Foster, E. M., Justice, A. W. and Matthews, V. (1978). Management of the demented elderly patient in the community. *Br. J. Psychiat.*, **132**, 441
Berkmann, L. F. and Syme, S. L. (1979). Social networks, host resistance and

mortality: a nine year follow-up of Alameda County residents. *Am. J. Epidemiol.*, **109**, 186

Challis, D. J., Chessum, R., Chesterman, J., Luckett, R. and Woods, B. (1987). Community Care for the frail elderly: an urban experiment. *Br. J. Social Wk*, **17**, 4; Supplement, 13

Challis, D. J. and Chesterman, J. (1985). A system for monitoring social work activity with the frail elderly. *Br. J. Social Wk*, **15**, 115

Challis, D. J. and Chesterman, J. (1986). Devolution to fieldworkers. *Social Services Insight*, 14 June, 15

Challis, D. J. and Chesterman, J. (1987). Feedback to front-line staff from computerised records: Some problems and progress. *Computer Applns Social Wk*, **3** (3), 12

Challis, D. J. and Davies, B. P. (1985). Long term care for the elderly: the Community Care Scheme. *Br. J. Social Wk*, **15**, 563

Challis, D. J. and Davies, B. P. (1986). *Case-management in Community Care.* Gower Press, Aldershot

Davies, B. P. and Challis, D. J. (1981). A production relations evaluation of the meeting of needs in the Community Care Projects. In Goldberg, E. M. and Connelly, N. (Eds.), *Evaluative Research in Social Care.* Heinemann, London

Davies, B. P. and Challis, D. J. (1986). *Matching Resources to Needs in Community Care.* Gower Press, Aldershot

Foster, E. M., Kay, D. W. K. and Bergmann, K. (1976). The characteristics of old people receiving and needing domiciliary services: the relevance of diagnoses. *Age and Ageing*, **5**, 245

Goldberg, D. P. and Huxley, P. (1980). *Mental Illness in the Community.* Tavistock, London

Goldberg, E. M. and Warburton, R. W. (1979). *Ends and Means in Social Work.* Allen and Unwin, London

Hall, M. R. P. (1982). Risk and health care. In Brearley, C. P. (Ed.), *Risk and Ageing.* Routledge, London

Hemsi, L. (1980). Psychogeriatric care in the community. *Hlth Trends*, **12**, 25

Hendriksen, C., Lund, E. and Strongard, E. (1984). Consequences of assessment and intervention among elderly people: a three year randomised controlled trial. *Br. Med. J.*, **289**, 1522

Luker, K. A. (1981). Health visiting and the elderly. *Nursing Times*, **77**, 137

Ratna, L. and Davies, J. (1984). Family therapy with the elderly mentally ill: some strategies and techniques. *Br. J. Psychiat.*, **145**, 311

Stevenson, O. and Parsloe, P. (1978). *Social Services' Teams: The Practitioner's View.* HMSO, London

Vetter, N. J., Jones, D. and Victor, C. (1984). Effect of health visitors working with elderly patients in general practice: a randomised controlled trial. *Br. Med. J.*, **288**, 369

Wattis, J. (1986). Abstracts: Medicine in society. *Ageing and Society*, **6**, 209

Yawney, B. and Slover, D. L. (1973). Relocation and the elderly. *Social Wk*, 18 May, 86

14
Living Environments for the Elderly.
1: Living at Home

Muir Gray

INTRODUCTION

Discussions of life at home often focus quickly on the professional services provided for old people in their own homes, but only a proportion of older people are dependent on intensive home support, and in this chapter I propose to discuss more fundamental issues related to life at home — namely, the objectives of good health at home, the types of intervention which can achieve these objectives, the patterns of care which can deliver these interventions, and the evaluation of health at home.

GOOD OBJECTIVES FOR GOOD HEALTH

Too often services for elderly people lack clear objectives, and set out below is a set of objectives for good health at home.

- To slow down the functional decline that occurs in old age. Some functional decline is inevitable, but for most people the rate of decline is greater than the rate of decline that would occur were ageing the only process affecting the individual. Loss of fitness leads to a gap between actual and potential levels of ability — the fitness gap (Figure 14.1) — and life at home, by encouraging and enabling activity, helps minimise the fitness gap and slow down the rate of functional decline (Gray *et al.*, 1985).
- To maintain and improve the quality of life in old age. Most older people would like to live on in their own homes, provided that they can be given sufficient support to do so, and the independence of life at home, coupled with the privacy of this setting, helps older people maintain a good quality of life.

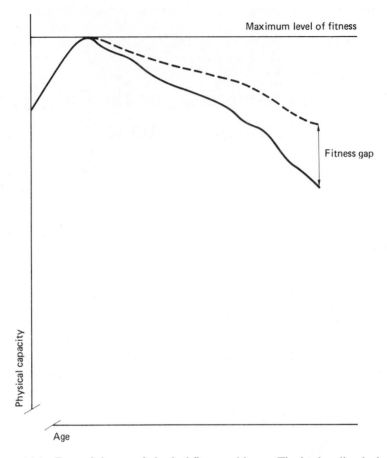

Figure 14.1   Rate of change of physical fitness with age. The broken line is the rate of decline due to ageing alone if fitness is not lost. The continuous line is the actual rate of decline. Source: Gray (1982)

- To provide support for the informal carers of older people. In Britain it was never common for elderly people to move in with their children as they grew older and more disabled. Living near, but not with, was the norm, and this should continue to be our objective. Many families find it impossible to care for older relatives if they have them in their own homes, because of the tensions that arise, whereas if housing policy were more flexible and allowed elderly people to move across country more easily to live near relatives, family support could be strengthened.
- To keep older people at home as long as possible. This may seem rather obvious but it is necessary to set out this objective in a discussion of life at home, because many services do not have the clear objective to

support life at home, although they may be very well-intentioned. Having set such an objective, one is able to define an explicit standard for home care and monitor its impact. For example, a standard for home care would be that no old person should be admitted to residential care until he or she had been offered at least three visits a day on a Saturday and Sunday, and such a standard would be easy to monitor by reviewing the cases of those admitted to residential care.

- To help older people have a good death as well as a good life. The quality of the last days of life is as important as the quality of the preceding years, and many older people would prefer to die in their own homes rather than in the impersonal surroundings of a hospital, provided that they could be given adequate support and assured of relief from distressing symptoms.

These are the objectives for good health at home. The interventions that can achieve these objectives are discussed in the next section.

EFFECTIVE INTERVENTIONS

An Adequate Income — The First Foundation

Any discussion of the support that is needed for elderly people at home must start with the provision of an adequate income. Many elderly people have an income that is too low to allow them to exist with comfort and confidence at home. There are a number of reasons for the low levels of income among elderly people:

- The low level of the State pension.
- The low number of people who are old at present who have a substantial occupational pension.
- Low rates of uptake of State benefits for which application must be made.
- A low rate of realisation and utilisation of capital.
- A low uptake of cost-saving opportunities such as double glazing or bulk buying.

In general, women are less well off than men, in part because of the higher prevalence of occupational pensions among men.

The Reasons for Poverty

The principal reason for the poverty of elderly people is, of course, the decision made by society that its resources should be provided more generously for those who are in work. There is no law of nature which lays down that the salary of a doctor, derived from taxation, should be several times higher than an old age pension, which is also derived from taxation. The fact that the former is considered to be doing useful work, whereas the latter has done useful work, is an arbitrary distinction but one that is perpetuated by consensus.

It is, perhaps, more fruitful to examine those attitudes and beliefs held by older people which perpetuate their own income and make life at home difficult.

The first is a fear of debt, related among some older people to fear of the workhouse — namely, compulsory institutionalisation. But the fear and dislike of debt goes much deeper than this, and debt, even an overdraft or a mortgage, is regarded as immoral by some older people.

Second, housebound older people often find it difficult to keep up with inflation and compare the price of goods as they are now with the cost of goods which they remembered in times past, and are unwilling to purchase some food or fuel or new clothes, because they are unable to appreciate that their income has kept up with inflation. For some elderly people decimalisation also still presents an additional problem which makes them reluctant to spend money.

Reducing the Prevalence of Poverty

In this section I shall not concentrate on the political moves which should be taken to reform the pension system in the United Kingdom but shall focus on steps that can be taken ideally to improve uptake of benefits, the realisation of capital, and the uptake of cost-saving opportunities.

- *Better-informed professionals* It is essential that the professionals who meet elderly people and whose opinion is trusted by elderly people — for example, district nurses, home helps and general practitioners — should know about the benefits that are available in the broadest terms and also know about the sources of advice and help for elderly people who wish to improve their income. It is not necessary for these workers to know the details of social security or annuity schemes, but they have to know they exist and use their relationship with the older person to provide him or her with the necessary emotional support to take what is, for many older people, a major step of exposing their financial problems to others and asking for help.
- *Better use of information services* Those who meet elderly people should concentrate more on putting them in touch with sources of expert advice such as the Citizens' Advice Bureau or a local bank.

Some primary care teams have developed a network of volunteers — for example, a retired bank manager — to facilitate this type of activity.

- *Better orientation of the financial services*   Banks and building societies should be encouraged to consider their response to the challenge of the ageing population. They should see old people not only as a group who need help, but also as a group with a considerable amount of capital who need financial advice.

The Provision of Appropriate Housing

Older people have a number of difficulties associated with their housing, the more common of which are:

- Difficulties with maintaining and repairing their dwelling.
- Difficulties with moving about their dwelling or getting in and out of it.
- Difficulties with heating.
- Anxiety and depression because of the environment in which they live.
- Inability to move to live nearer relatives.
- Lack of basic amenities.

The reasons for these problems may be divided into two different groups — those related to the low income levels of older people and those related to disability.

Focusing on the former, many of the housing problems of older people could be solved if they had a reasonable level of income. The older person who has, for example, an income the same as that of a doctor is able to resolve many of the problems listed above, although he or she may require expert help to do so if disability should develop. An old person who is well-off can move from one county to another because he or she can afford to purchase a flat or bungalow in the desired area. In addition, such people can improve and repair their dwelling and keep it warm, whereas elderly persons with a low income are relatively powerless.

Similarly, the onset of disability creates many problems for older people with regard to housing. For example, a house that is perfectly suitable for a person when fit and active may become completely unsuitable when a stroke or other disabling disease creates an inability to climb a flight of stairs. Similarly, the onset of a chronic disabling disease such as heart disease or chronic lung disease increases the vulnerability of older people to cold, and there is now good evidence that we should aim for a minimum temperature of 16 °C in the rooms used by elderly people (Mant and Gray, 1986).

Furthermore, disability compounds the difficulties that older people have in solving their problems, for it is much more difficult to visit the building society, Environmental Health Department or the rates rebate office when one is disabled.

The Prevention of Disease

The prevention of disease in youth and middle age has an important impact on health in old age, but there is also considerable scope for prevention after the age of 65 has been reached. The types of disease that can be prevented in old age are listed in Table 14.1. Some of these diseases are prevented by

Table 14.1   Scope for disease prevention in old age. Source: Gray (1982)

Iatrogenic disease
Depression
Anxiety
Alcoholism
Hypothermia
Influenza
Tetanus
Constipation
Some types of fall
Some types of incontinence
Malnutrition

specific medical interventions, others by broader social and environmental measures. Furthermore, loss of fitness can be prevented and life at home maintained. Promoting self-care has a major part to play in the loss of fitness and will be discussed in the next main section.

The Effective Management of Acute Illness

Because elderly people have difficulties in gaining access to medical services — for example, because of the low prevalence of telephone and car ownership — and because they are, in general, unwilling to make demands of the general practitioner, acute illness in old age may not be presented to the primary care team as quickly as is the case with people of younger age. Furthermore, the primary care team may not respond as quickly to illness in old age as it does to illness in childhood, for example, although elderly people are at least as vulnerable as young people to the adverse effects of acute episodes of illness. To ensure that an old person continues to live at home in good health, it is, therefore, essential for primary care teams to try to provide a much more effective service for the management of acute illness, and this would range from education of elderly people as to when to consult, through to ensuring that new receptionists are informed of the importance of relaying apparently insignificant telephone calls from elderly people to the general practitioner as quickly as possible. Furthermore, general practitioners need to improve their competence in dealing with conditions such as acute confusional states (Almind *et al.*, 1985).

More Effective Management of Chronic Illness

Most elderly people with chronic disabling disease live at home, and the effective management of chronic disabling disease by slowing the rate of decline can have an important bearing on the length of time an older person may be able to live at home and on the quality of life in this setting.

The Provision of Support to Families and Other Informal Carers

Life at home for many older people is dependent upon the support they receive from family, friends, neighbours and volunteers, and it is essential that these informal carers receive support if they are to continue to intervene effectively.

TYPES OF CARE

Self-care

Self-care is the most important type of care for elderly people living at home, for two reasons.

First, it is quantitatively the most significant type of care, a fact over-looked by many professionals. We talk glibly of very dependent people being supported at home, or severely disabled older people receiving intensive home care; but when such cases are examined, it becomes obvious that the amount of professional assistance they are receiving covers not more than two or three hours in the day. For the remaining 21 hours of the day the disabled elderly person is coping on his or her own. Without self-care professional care would be ineffective in maintaining older people in their own homes.

Second, self-care is so important because of the need to promote physical fitness and well-being in old age. As described in the opening paragraph of this chapter, many of the changes that occur in old age and which were formerly ascribed to the ageing process (Table 14.2) are in fact due to decades of inactivity. Because of the effects of the ageing process, inactivity has probably a greater impact on older people than on young people, and if elderly people are not given the opportunity to continue to practise a particular skill, then they will lose it, and all four aspects of fitness — strength, stamina, suppleness and skill — can be very easily lost

Table 14.2 Changes commonly assumed to be the result of normal ageing but which have been observed in young people or those experiencing weightlessness. Source: Bortz (1982)

Decrease in	Increase in
V_{O_2max}	Systolic blood pressure
Cardiac output	Peripheral resistance
Stroke volume	Intolerance to tilting
Plasma volume	
Lean body mass	
Bone density	
Insulin sensitivity	

with inactivity. Obviously, there is a need to promote physical activity in old age and encourage older people to take up swimming or dancing or music and movement. Yet the most important type of therapy is the occupational therapy and physiotherapy of everyday life. Too often, older people are offered prostheses to take over the functions they have lost, instead of the therapy they need to help them regain the functions they have lost.

This means that we must review the contribution of many services that we have traditionally held in high esteem, services such as the meals-on-wheels service or the home help service. The danger in these prosthetic services is that they are given to people who could be helped to regain the skills that have been lost, but because referral is to a social agency rather than a health agency, the people receiving the referral are not in a position to question the need for the prosthesis. In some cases the need for meals-on-wheels is obvious, as when, for example, the principal supporter of an older person has become ill and been admitted to hospital, but if the request for meals-on-wheels is simply because an older person is failing to cope, somebody should ask the question, 'Why is this old person failing to cope?' This approach is increasingly adopted when an older person is deemed to be in need of residential care, because Brocklehurst *et al.* (1978) demonstrated that a proportion of people deemed to be in need of residential care had remediable health problems, but it now needs to be applied much more widely.

Ageism and Protectionism

Simply arguing that we should develop a particular service because it has biological benefits is unlikely to achieve change unless we take into account the social and psychological context in which these services are offered and received.

First, it should be said that most older people are keen to maintain their abilities and regain lost skills, as a recent study (MacHeath, 1984) into the attitudes of older people towards physical exercise has demonstrated.

Second, it must be remembered that many older people who are given home care services such as the visit of a nursing auxiliary or meals-on-wheels during a time of illness find it very hard to relinquish that service, because of the personal relationship that develops with the person delivering it and the isolation that will result if the visiting stops. Independence is invariably seen as desirable by providers of services, for it reduces demands on the service, but to the housebound older person independence in some particular aspect of life may make the quality of life worse by increasing isolation. Often the old person is aware that the struggle to achieve an increase in functional ability will result in the loss of the treasured home help or nursing auxiliary without the achievement of sufficient improvement to get back to the shops or the church or the pub.

It is the beliefs and attitudes of other people which present more of a problem in the promotion of self-care. Many people believe that all older people are affected principally by the ageing process, and are therefore unable to change or learn or develop in any way. This ageist belief inevitably leads to a prosthetic approach to service provision. In addition, and probably more difficult to overcome, is the guilt that is felt by many people about the plight of older people in our society — a guilt which generates not desire to change the lot of older people but a desire to cosset and comfort elderly people, providing them with tokens of esteem rather than the means to lead an independent and healthy life. Some of the services which are provided for older people do as much to allay the anxiety of society at large as to help older people achieve their full potential, and they allay the feelings of guilt of those who are well-off about the plight of those whom they see as less privileged, though no less deserving, than themselves (Gray, 1981).

In this context, it is important to remember that professionals are not immune from this attitude and that professionals often speak of elderly people as being dependent on them, whereas *they* are, in fact, dependent upon the severely disabled older person. It is in the interests of the professions to perpetuate the image of older people as a disabled, demanding, dependent group whose need is for more highly paid professional helpers. It will require considerable confidence and maturity for professionals to change the image of older people and see that there will be just as great a need for professional support in a new style of practice based on therapeutic and educational principles as in the old style, in which older people are seen as a passive dependent group waiting to receive the benefits of professional intervention.

Informal Care

The second most important type of care is informal care — that given by friends, neighbours, family and voluntary associations.

The contribution made by friends and neighbours is often underestimated by professional helpers, and sometimes under-represented by the elderly person. It is true that in some inner-city areas elderly people live in a hostile social environment, but many elderly people receive a great deal of help from friends and neighbours. The probability that an old person will receive support from these sources is, of course, a function of the personality of the old person, and older people who are less rewarding — for example, because they complain frequently — may exhaust the goodwill of friends and neighbours and be referred for professional help earlier than the old person who is always interested in other people and grateful for the help he or she receives.

Insensitive professional intervention can disrupt informal networks assistance, and care should be taken, before initiating a service such as meals-on-wheels, to identify the precise pattern of informal care which is at present supporting the old person.

Changes in family size and structure (for example, the earlier age of marriage of women and the decrease in family size), combined with an increase in population mobility, have reduced the opportunities which families have to provide support for elderly relatives. There is, however, no evidence that the provision of State support has reduced the willingness of families to care.

Many professionals, of course, observe an increase in the number of families who are unwilling to care for elderly relatives, but the total number of families caring for elderly people has increased considerably over the same period of time.

Each family has its breaking point, and the rate at which this point is reached depends on two variables. The first is the nature of the relationship between the old person and his or her family. The old person who was a good and loving parent, always keen to sacrifice for the children, is more likely to be supported for longer than the old person who was exacting or demanding or unfair as a parent; when children leave home, they are mostly in debt to their parents, but the size of that debt varies from family to family. The rate at which parental credit was used up also varies from family to family, depending upon the rate of decline of the older person and on the support provided for the family.

Many family problems could be prevented if elderly people were helped to move near their children rather than being forced to live with them, as is the case with those elderly people who have insufficient resources to buy a dwelling themselves. A more flexible approach to housing mobility in old age would help many older people move to live near their family and thus reduce the tension within the family.

It therefore emerges that three types of measure can be taken to prevent family breakdown:

- *Measures to slow the rate of decline*   The better the clinical care of the older person, the slower will be the rate of decline and the less will be the demands on the family.
- *Measures to provide support for the carer*   If the carer is given practical support (for example, by the provision of meals-on-wheels to free him or her from the daily tie of the elderly parent, or home help or financial help), the strain is reduced and the ability of the carer to support the old person will be prolonged. Sometimes the relatives need support to modify the behaviour of the older person, and although there is scope for therapeutic work with families looking after elderly relatives, in most cases the relationships have been so strongly established for so long that the carer must be given either simple support or very practical behavioural techniques to modify distressing behaviour.
- *Measures to provide relief for the carer*   Carers need relief, whether in the form of relief for the day or for the night or for longer periods of time. As important as the provision of periods of relief is the establishment of a clear understanding between the carer and the professional supporters about the way in which care will be shared. Rather than simply telling the family that they will be offered support when needed, a firm commitment to the planned provision of regular periods of respite can not only provide practical relief from the burden of caring, but also minimise anxiety by relieving the family from the need to decide when to seek additional help.

Domiciliary Care

Much has been written already about the ways in which domiciliary care can be developed, but it is perhaps more important to emphasise the principles of professional practice which should permeate domiciliary care much more strongly than they do at present. Enid Levin and her colleagues (1983) carried out a survey of the supporters of elderly people with mental infirmity, and found that although relatives would like extra resources to be provided, they were very concerned about the style of professional help they had been given. Relatives had found it supportive to have professionals who (Levin *et al.*, 1983):

- arranged interviews promptly;
- made it clear who they were, where they came from and why they were visiting;
- showed sensitivity in their dealings with the elderly person;

- were willing to listen to the supporters and showed concern about their well-being;
- gave clear explanations;
- understood the possible causes of confusion;
- where a diagnosis of dementia was made, through careful questioning, established the precise problems which its management posed;
- agreed a clear and promptly implemented plan of action.

Because the present pattern of domiciliary services and the present mixture of professionals has developed in a piecemeal and disjointed fashion over the last century, it is not surprising that they bear little relationship to the actual needs of older people: consider, for example, how many bits of the governmental machine are involved in the fine task of helping older people keep warm in their own homes. It is, therefore, important to look for ways in which the barriers imposed by bureaucratic and professional structures can be minimised.

One approach is to try to develop service planning for small populations of older people, thus reducing the number of professionals who have to get to know and trust one another.

A second approach is to provide the elderly person with sufficient information about the various types of help being received, so that he or she can act as a link between the various professional services.

A third approach is to set clear objectives, either for the population of older people or for the individual old person, so that the professionals will focus less on interprofessional disputes as their gaze is focused outwards on the health problems of older people.

Hospital and Institutional Care

It is ridiculous to use the term 'community care' to mean care outside hospital, for this implies that the hospital is not a community service, which is patently absurd (Gray, 1983). Accordingly, it is necessary to move away from the two-box model of care, which concentrates on two types of professional care, to a four-box model of care, which describes the present position more accurately (Figure 14.2).

In the development of services it is, therefore, essential to promote an integrated pattern of care based on self-care and informal care instead of focusing on a rather sterile debate about the shift from 'hospital' to 'community care'.

The principles developed by the World Health Organization for primary health care planning are increasingly used as a basis for service development, because of their simplicity and validity:

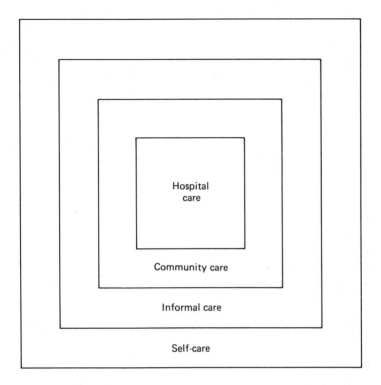

Figure 14.2   The four-box system of health care

- Services should be delivered to the whole population.
- There should be participation of elderly people, both individually and collectively, in the development of a service.
- There should be an effective and efficient use of resources, with appropriate use of technology.
- There should be strong collaboration between all relevant agencies.

All of these principles are equally important, but perhaps the most challenging is the exhortation to promote the participation of elderly people both individually and collectively in the development of services provided for them.

EVALUATION

In part because of the anxiety generated by the ageing of the population, relatively little attention has been given to evaluation of services for older people and that which has been given to it has resulted in the production of data which focus on the structure and process of service delivery rather than on the outcome. The main challenge for the future is the development of outcome measures that could be used by people managing services who do not have the types of resources which research workers have when carrying out research projects which include service evaluation.

Until the services for elderly people are able to set clear objectives and measure progress or the lack of it, professionals will continue to react to the challenge of the ageing population less effectively and less efficiently than they could do were they to work with older people to meet the challenge in a coherent and thoughtful fashion.

REFERENCES

Almind, G., Freer, C., Gray, J. A. M. and Warshaw, G. (1985). The contribution of the primary care doctor to the medical care of the elderly in the community. *Dan. Med. Bull.*, Special Supplement Series, No. 2: *Gerontology*

Bortz, W. M. (1982). Disuse and aging. *J. Am. Med. Ass.*, **248**, 1203

Brocklehurst, J. C., Leeming, J. T., Carty, M. H. and Robinson, J. M. (1978). Medical screening of old people accepted for residential care, *Lancet*, **2**, 141

Gray, J. A. M. (1981). Do we care too much for our elders? *Lancet*, **1**, 1289

Gray, J. A. M. (1982). Practising prevention in old age. *Br. Med. J.*, **285**, 545

Gray, J. A. M. (1983). Four box health care development in a time of zero growth. *Lancet*, 19 November, 1185

Gray, J. A. M., Bassey, E. J. and Young, A. (1985). The risks of inactivity. In Gray, J. A. M. (Ed.), *Prevention of Disease in the Elderly*, pp. 78–94. Churchill Livingstone, Edinburgh

Levin, E., Sinclair, I. and Gorbach, P. (1983). *The Supporters of Confused Elderly People at Home*. National Institute for Social Work, London

MacHeath, J. A. (1984). *Activity, Health and Fitness in Old Age*. Croom Helm, London

Mant, D. and Gray, J. A. M. (1986). *Building Regulations and Health* (Report for the Building Research Establishment). Department of the Environment, London

15
Living Environments for the Elderly. 2: Promoting the 'Right' Institutional Environment

Sheila Peace

INTRODUCTION

The vast majority of older people live in a wide variety of ordinary housing in the community. In contrast, residential homes, nursing homes and hospitals accommodate approximately 6 per cent of the elderly population (Tinker, 1984). However, with advanced age the possibility of living in such settings increases, and among this group are some of the most frail and vulnerable members of society. The average age of residents in residential homes is in the mid-eighties, and data from the 1981 Census show that, for England and Wales, whereas only 2–3 per cent of those of pensionable age were living permanently in residential establishments, the proportion rises to 13 per cent for those over 85 years, a figure which also shows wide regional variation (Office of Population Censuses and Surveys, 1983; Peace, 1986a). To some extent, these figures reflect societal changes which may make institutional living a more commonplace experience for a minority of the very old. Such changes include the growing number of the 'old' old within an ageing population, who are potentially more 'at risk'; fluctuations in employment/unemployment and its effect on family care for the elderly, particularly among women; present government support for the growth of private residential and nursing home care; patterns of retirement migration; and the increase in specialised housing for older people, which may result in a greater acceptance of alternative living environments in later life (Peace, 1986a).

At present it is too early to predict the outcome of these changes. However, such developments have reopened the debate concerning the nature and role of institutional environments both present and future, even though institutional living cannot be said to be a 'preferred option' for most

217

old people. The main theme of this chapter therefore focuses on whether we can promote the 'right' institutional environment. In doing so, it examines the relationship between domestic and institutional environments; considers past and present attempts to remodel residential settings; and draws on the views of the consumer in looking at what type of living environment might be most acceptable in future. While discussion is based primarily on experiences within residential homes, it is felt that such comments have direct application for nursing environments. Throughout the text short vignettes capturing the lives of three old people are used to highlight the realities of living in different types of environment. The three vignettes are part fact, part fiction, based on people and settings encountered by the author in her research into elderly people and their environments.

First, we must ask how realistic it is for the institutional setting to try and compensate for or replace the loss of one's own home, and to do this we need to know more about the home life of old people.

THE IMPORTANCE OF HOME

Mrs E lives in a small semidetached council house on an interwar estate. She has lived there over thirty years and has spent the last ten years alone since her husband died. Now in her eighties, she no longer goes out of the house unaided, as she finds it difficult to walk far, owing to arthritic legs and a heart complaint. Her brother, who lives locally, does most of her shopping and she can always call on a neighbour if necessary. She receives meals-on-wheels three days a week and manages to cook at least one hot meal on other days. The house is small: at the front door you are confronted with a room on your left — the bathroom; a room on your right — the living-room with kitchen adjacent; and in front of you steep steps leading to two bedrooms. For the past three years Mrs E has slept in the living-room; her single bed placed next to the front window surrounded by a sofa, two armchairs, the television, a small table and a large sideboard covered in photos of her daughter and grandchildren and stacked high with books, magazines and letters. She is not an early riser, and may make tea and go back to bed with the paper. She likes to burn a coal fire in the kitchen, where she spends most of the morning, but in the afternoon she sits in the living-room by the electric fire and reads or watches TV. She does not have many visitors — her daughter lives abroad — but those who do come, come every week: her brother, the district nurse, a student from the local college, a neighbour, and at least once a week she's picked up by ambulance and taken to a local club. She talks of getting a cat. While she sometimes says that she feels frustrated and lonely, she would hate to leave her home, and if the subject is raised, will talk of friends who have 'gone into a home' as 'on their way out'.

Research has shown that residents of old people's homes are predominantly widowed females in their early to mid-eighties, and that a large proportion have lived alone prior to admission (Willcocks *et al.*, 1982; Weaver *et al.*, 1985). The reasons for entering a residential home are varied and complex: some people are admitted after a stay in hospital; others find that ill-health, coupled with either their own inability to cope alone or a carer's inability to cope, make a residential place an attractive proposition. But whatever the reason for admission to care, most will have spent a lifetime in their own home. Data also show that, of those old people aged 80 years and over living in the community, more than half live alone and hardly any live with those who are not relatives (Willcocks *et al.*, 1986). A major contrast between living at home and living in a home is, therefore, 'living with strangers' and surrendering one's personal privacy.

In our society the conceptualisation of home is intimately bound up with family. Home is essentially a private place — the centre of domesticity but also a place for intimacy, for solitude, a place from which to gain strength to engage in the public sphere (Willcocks *et al.*, 1986). It can also be viewed from a number of perspectives — physical or material, social and psychological. In the physical sense, home is a place where we are in control, where we can permit or deny access. It is a defensible space. The acquisition of objects within the home may encourage a level of possessiveness, but also enables us to develop a familiarity with our environment which is reinforced through memories that help us to connect the past with the present. As a social setting, home means people and their relationships. Although older people may live alone and experience a reduced social network, it can be argued that they can still retain links with their community, albeit at second hand, which enable them to maintain an important sense of self-identity (Howell, 1983; Rowles, 1983). Here the social and psychological facets of home converge and we begin to catch a glimpse of the meaning of home for older people. It is often said that older people are attached to their homes, and this attachment is shown in both their unusually long residence in a single location and the desire of a majority for living out their lives at home. Studies of older people's satisfaction with their housing point to the complexity of the topic: people want to stay put because home has associations with family and related memories, particularly true for older women, for whom home is very much their domain; they feel competent in a familiar environment where disability may appear unremarkable; if home-owners, the status of ownership gives them a sense of control in a world which devalues them, and they find that they can trade-off some of the costs of remaining at home by recognising some of the comforts (Golant, 1982; O'Bryant, 1983; Sixsmith, 1986).

The words 'competence', 'value', 'status' all point to the importance of home as a power base for old people, and it is, perhaps, useful at this point to draw upon the work of psychologists from the field of environment and ageing to help us gain a fuller understanding of what we mean here. Two concepts are particularly useful — environmental congruence and environmental press. During the course of our lives, we adapt our environment to meet our needs — that is, we remain in congruence — but there are also times when our needs are out of tune with our environment. Such environmental press can occur for many reasons: we may not have the material resources to enable us to adapt our surroundings; the circumstances of ownership of property may not allow for adaptation; or we may not be physically competent to make such adaptations and help may not be readily available. Lawton and colleagues have conceptualised this process in what is called the 'environmental docility hypothesis' — that is, the less competent the individual the greater the impact of environmental factors on that individual (Lawton and Nahemow, 1973; Lawton, 1980). At a crude level, then, we might use this concept to suggest that older people with increasingly frail health require a more supportive environment. But Lawton's definition of competence is complex, involving not only biological health, but also cognitive skill and ego strength (Lawton, 1983). He also suggests that a certain level of environmental press can create a tension through which the individual may experience growth. This may explain why it seems that many older people choose to go on living at home in accommodation which for a variety of reasons could be considered stressful, while those in institutional settings often appear to sink into apathy and inactivity.

To summarise, then: We have noted that a majority of the very old live in ordinary housing in the community. For many their environment will be familiar, offering privacy and enabling them to achieve a level of competence within familiar surroundings. While the physical environment may not be ideal, compensations may exist in terms of the maintenance of self-identity. With this picture in mind, we can now consider what we know of institutional living environments for older people, and try to understand whether or not it is possible for such settings to compensate for a loss of home.

THE CHARACTERISTICS OF INSTITUTIONS

For many authors the institution has been viewed as a form of social control that masquerades as social care (see Jones and Fowles, 1984). The routine surveillance of residents imposes control over all aspects of their lives — time, space, movement — and this commonly results in a loss of autonomy, responsibility and self-identity. The manifestation of such traits is perhaps best described in Goffman's seminal essays on 'total institutions'

(1961). In presenting an abstracted ideal of the institution against which reality can be measured, he identifies four main characteristics of institutional living: the rigidity of routine; the block treatment of residents/ patients; the depersonalisation of residents/patients; and the social distance between staff and residents. These themes have been developed by researchers working within a range of settings (Wing and Brown, 1970; King *et al.*, 1971), and many authors have commented on the outcome for resident/ patient behaviour: the enforced apathy; the loss of contact with the outside world; the loss of personal possessions and personal events; the feelings of submissiveness and resignation; and the development of relationships which appear superficial and unsatisfactory (Townsend and Kimbell, 1975; Raynes *et al.*, 1979).

Such characteristics offer a direct contrast with those of the home life of old people outlined above. While it may be argued that residential settings for old people do not present such an extreme form of institutional living as that portrayed in the psychiatric hospital or prison, and that the frail elderly may require a level of support from staff which makes a degree of surveillance necessary, the themes of privacy, autonomy and choice all remain key factors of residential life for old people. It is to that life that I now turn.

INSTITUTIONAL SETTINGS: PAST AND PRESENT

Miss G is a tall, thin, silent woman in her late seventies living in a residential home. Before entering the home, she had lived with her elder sister in a small terraced house in a neighbouring district some four miles away. Her own health is poor; she has in the past ten years undergone a mastectomy for breast cancer, and her sister had undertaken most of the household tasks. Her sister's death two years ago had therefore left her both bereft and with few resources to draw upon. She found herself agreeing to come into the home, as it seemed the only solution to her situation. The home is a large establishment with 60 residents, set in spacious grounds — bordered on one side by a railway line and on the other by the backs of private houses. Although only a quarter of a mile from the local shopping centre, the home appears isolated. The building is E-shaped, on two floors, and each fork of the E is a separate block with one four-bedded room, one double bedroom and four single bedrooms. The back of the E contains the dining-room, kitchen and administrative areas. Miss G shares a double room on Block C. Her room is sparsely furnished: two beds, side by side; two bedside lockers, two chests, two wardrobes, two hardbacked chairs, one washbasin. The floor is covered with green linoleum and the beds have matching pink candlewick bedspreads.

There are very few personal belongings in the room. Her room-mate has a few pictures of her family arranged on her locker, but Miss G has nothing except her washbag and a comb on top of the chest. Life in the home revolves around communal routines. Breakfast is served in the central dining-room at 8.30 a.m., lunch at 12.30 p.m., tea at 4.30 p.m. Bath times are organised on a weekly rota and staff go about their duties to a predetermined schedule. Miss G spends most of her day sitting in the lounge in Block C; she does not read or chat, she just stares into space. No one knows very much about Miss G.

Those involved in trying to bring about changes in our nursing and residential homes for older people sometimes express the view that we should try and forget the past, adopt a new attitude and promote a positive image for the future. While these are laudable sentiments, it is only by a study of the evolution of institutional settings that we can begin to understand their characteristics and decide whether or not we can promote an alternative form of environment.

In the past, institutions were founded to accommodate the indigent poor, the mentally ill, the 'work-shy': those people seen as marginal to society. Among these were many elderly people, and although it is true that both the private and voluntary sectors provided such accommodation in the nineteenth century, the extent of such provision was small, and most people were housed in the public workhouse (later known as public assistance institutions). The prime function of the workhouse system was containment rather than care, and the harsh realities of such communal living are well documented (Townsend, 1962; Peace, 1986b). The legacy of the institutional past, therefore, has little to do with the development of housing for all, the family dwelling unit and home-ownership (Swenarton, 1981): the one focusing on the needs of the family, stressing the virtues of privacy and 'independent' living; the other, on the containment of those who somehow did not fit society's norms.

It was not until the welfare reforms following World War II that the first legislation regarding residential homes was enacted. Thus Section 21 of the *National Assistance Act 1948* placed a duty on all local authorities to provide 'residential accommodation for persons who by reason of age, infirmity or any other circumstances are in need of care and attention not otherwise available to them'. In many respects this legislation confirmed the role of the State in providing for those either without family or whose family could not support them. In terms of provision, many local authorities had to continue to make do with workhouse accommodation during the post-war period, but others followed the call for a small-scale hotel model and began to use old adapted properties which accommodated 30–35 residents. Later, however, economies of scale led to an increase in larger purpose-built homes for 40–60 residents (Means and Smith, 1983; Peace, 1986b).

The development of new-build accommodation prompted a succession of guidance from central government concerning the physical environment of homes (Department of Health and Social Security and Welsh Office, 1962, 1973), and it is interesting to note that it is within such design guidance that we see evidence of official concern with the nature of institutions. A series of issues emerged which have remained central to the debate about the nature of change in such settings. These include the analogy with the domestic setting — the need for the residential homes to fulfil the functions of the domestic home; the associated demand for increased personal privacy; and the importance of community integration as a reaction to the often enforced isolation of institutions in the past. However, alongside such official publications, authors such as Townsend (1962) alerted us to the continuing harsh realities of institutional living, and during the late 1960s and 1970s a series of reports concerning the quality of life for elderly people within institutional settings called for greater attention to be paid to the underlying philosophy of care and the need for greater resident autonomy, choice over lifestyle and personal privacy — aspects of daily living that are common facets of life at home (Peace, 1986b). The time was right, therefore, for a reassessment of the nature of institutional living for old people.

RESIDENTIAL LIVING IN THE 1980s

How far are we justified in maintaining that the characteristics of institutionalisation outlined above still persist within institutional settings for old people in the 1980s? In order to explore some of these issues, data are used from two studies of residential homes carried out by the Centre for Environmental and Social Studies in Ageing at the Polytechnic of North London since 1980. The first is the national consumer study in 100 Local Authority Homes (1980/81) and the second a smaller replication of this study within ten private residential homes in Norfolk (1982/83) (Willcocks *et al.*, 1982; Weaver *et al.*, 1985)*. The major issues of routinisation, loss of personal identity and the social distance between residents and staff are perhaps best explored in relation to three related themes — privacy, autonomy and surveillance, the first two building on the analogy of life within the domestic setting, and the third enabling us to consider something

---

* It should be noted that although both studies are called 'consumer studies', an important distinction can be made between the clients of public sector provision and the clients/ consumers of private sector provision, dependent upon whether a direct or indirect payment has been made for the service.

of the relationships and levels of responsibility that exist between residents and staff in residential settings.

The concept of privacy has many interpretations implying seclusion, solitude and even anonymity for both the individual and/or the individual and intimate others. The roles attached to domestic life, the family and home all have associations of privacy, but how far does privacy manifest itself within residential homes for old people? In the public sector, where old people's homes may commonly accommodate 40–50 residents in purpose-built property, opportunities for personal privacy are often controlled by both physical and organisational factors. In the National Consumer Study only half of all the residents in the 100 homes had a bedroom of their own; the rest shared, mainly with one or two others (Willcocks *et al.*, 1982). Thus, many residents were denied even potential access to a space in which they could enjoy a degree of personal seclusion. Yet the research showed that access to personal space encouraged social interaction: those residents with a room of their own made more friends.

Of course availability of a personal space does not convey the rights of ownership, and in many residential homes in the public sector the smooth operation of the organisation demands that residents live a predominantly public life — spending most of the day in large communal lounges or dining-rooms. This very public and communal lifestyle can be attributed to a range of staffing practices — staff numbers; shift working; and the centralisation of key services (cooking, cleaning, laundry, bathing) — as well as to the design of many homes. The maintenance of a private life for many residents therefore becomes impossible, and in this respect a level of depersonalisation may exist, characteristic of other institutional settings (Peace *et al.*, 1982; Willcocks *et al.*, 1986).

In contrast to local authority provision, to date, the private residential sector has capitalised on the image of providing small 'homely' family units embodied in the old adapted properties commonly used as homes. Yet the number of residents in private homes having a bedroom of their own appears to be no greater than in the public sector, even though bedroom space forms the major commodity to be purchased. For this reason, great emphasis is placed on the utilisation of private space, often at the expense of public areas. Examples from the Norfolk study showed how adapted properties had been extended to create additional bedrooms, while existing lounges/dining-rooms were maintained, often failing to accommodate a majority of residents (Weaver *et al.*, 1985). By default, therefore, some residents were forced to spend long periods of time, including mealtimes, in their rooms — a level of seclusion bordering on isolation that cannot really be equated with the freedom to choose personal privacy.

Of course, this discussion of privacy also raises issues concerning the levels of autonomy experienced by old people in residential settings: to what degree do residents experience freedom of action? Again the nature of both the physical and social/organisational environments places constraints on resident autonomy, and in the public and private sectors examples can be cited of the routinisation and lack of choice over everyday aspects of life, especially mealtimes, bathtimes, rising and retiring; the lack of activity; and the poor quality of the physical environment, which impedes mobility and environmental control. Although it would appear from our research that the nature of the experience for residents may vary within different types of setting, dependent both on the resources available and on the principles on which the home is run, there also appears to be an underlying uniformity which is difficult to overcome (see Booth, 1985; Willcocks *et al.*, 1986). At one extreme the weight of responsibility placed upon those who run homes may manifest itself in the routine surveillance of residents and an emphasis on physical care, while at the other a policy of minimum intervention by staff — again predominantly in the form of physical care — may result in a lifestyle for residents which, although purporting to respect resident individuality, results in an equally unsatisfactory style of care. To return to the earlier discussion of environmental congruence, we may find that neither style of management creates a setting in which the individual can experience personal growth through the support of others.

Thus, it would appear that some aspects of institutional living, whatever the setting, are always at odds with the model of domestic family living which appears to underpin so much of our thinking about residential care. The two are largely incompatible, and although it may be important for us to try to minimise the differences between domestic home and residential home, it often proves tokenistic to do so. A good example of such tokenism has been the attempt made in some local authority homes to establish small group living. In this model a home with 40 or 50 residents is split into four or five, often physically separate units, of 8–10 residents (Peace and Harding, 1980; Willcocks *et al.*, 1986). The idea is to create a surrogate family unit, and it is common for a staff member to be assigned as a key worker for the group. While research about group-living homes remains limited, there is some evidence that such strategies fail to create a family group, but instead only re-create features of the wider institution in miniature (Willcocks *et al.*, 1986). Although residents may benefit from an improved physical environment, their lives often continue to revolve around the routines of the large institution, with the additional pressures of having to cope with small-group interaction.

Much of the above discussion points to the fact that, whatever the setting, residential homes exhibit features of collective living which cannot be equated to private lives at home. Yet the recognition of the needs of a changing and ageing society forces us to face the question that if institutional living, for some elderly people, is here to stay, then how do we promote the 'right institutional' environment, one that offers the old person a positive experience of collective living while maintaining his or her individuality?

PROMOTING THE 'RIGHT' INSTITUTIONAL ENVIRONMENT

Mr P, a man in his mid-seventies, came to live at the Centre two years after the death of his wife. Although he had coped passably well living alone, a recent series of dizzy spells had resulted in a fall which had left him feeling low and vulnerable. He had known the Centre for some time. He'd watched it being built and had later come to take his lunchtime meals there at the restaurant-style lunch club. The Centre is really a small L-shaped complex of living accommodation and daytime services for older people. There are two types of accommodation, offering the same physical environment but different levels of social support. The more independent living unit occupies three floors of a four-storey block, each floor having ten bedsitting rooms, a communal lounge/diner and a well-equipped kitchen. The ground floor accommodates the large communal dining-room used for the lunch club, an adjacent kitchen, a small day centre and administrative offices. Next to this block is the two-storey residential unit, offering more supportive care. Mr P lives on the third floor of the independent living unit. His bedsitting room, like all the others, has been decorated by an interior designer. There is attractive pinewood furniture which is geared to the needs of older people, wallpaper with matching curtains and covers, and carpet on the floor. Mr P has made himself at home: he has installed his own portable television, a row of books line the shelf above his bed and a number of plants festoon the windowsills. The atmosphere is relaxed and yet communal routines do exist: residents who cannot manage to bathe unaided are helped; rooms are cleaned and laundry changed on particular days; and meals are available at set times in the lounge/diners. But somehow you don't notice the staff, and many residents structure their own time; they get up late and make their own breakfast; they go out, sit in their room or join a friend in the lounge. Mr P feels that he has made friends here and that he made the right decision to move.

In a recent review of a variety of institutional settings, the American gerontologist Robert Kastenbaum argues that a 'therapeutic environment will need to provide treatments, replacements and compensations' (Kastenbaum, 1983, p. 12). From the above discussion we would agree, perhaps, that living environments for old people, which are not their own home, have to incorporate a number of elements: the supportive care of staff, a prosthetic environment and a warm and friendly atmosphere. But is this the kind of environment that old people want? To date, we have very little information concerning the environmental preferences of the frail elderly. We know that some people would welcome a move to small ground-floor accommodation, while others like the security of knowing that staff are on hand. We also know that many people lack information concerning housing options and that a fear of institutional living still exists (Fengler *et al.*, 1985; Wheeler, 1985). In addition, we have been able to learn something of the advantages and disadvantages of shared living from small-scale experiments in alternative housing emerging in many Western developed countries — e.g. group homes, shared houses and apartments. Such initiatives tell us a great deal about the cultural constraints which delimit our own style of living and raise several questions as to how we create the appropriate balance between the familial and the bureaucratic environment; the individual and the communal setting; the expressive and the instrumental relationship of staff and residents (Peace with Nusberg, 1984). Indeed, success of many schemes appears to be due to 'the separateness afforded — i.e. privacy and independence — at least as much as to the availability of togetherness' (Bernard Liebowitz commenting on the community housing programme at the Philadelphia Geriatric Center — Liebowitz, 1978, p. 140).

Such sentiments would appear to be echoed by the residents of old people's homes in England, for data from the National Consumer Study in local authority homes showed that elderly residents wanted environmental control. They expressed a preference for a room of their own; windows they could open; temperature they could control; access to an ordinary bath — facets of daily living which the researchers identified as *normal, unexceptional and non-institutional*, and which they used as a guide for reconstructing the residential environment around the needs of the individual (Willcocks *et al.*, 1982). They state:

> Taking our cue from the choices made by old people, we must begin by identifying those features of existing arrangements which threaten their ability to achieve dignity and self-esteem. At a macro level we would wish to demonstrate explicitly to our clients and to those who care about their well-being that we are prepared to construct environments that are a worthy setting for our respected elders. We must assert, by the nature of the old age home, that it offers a meaningful life for people who are valued and cherished.
>
> (Willcocks *et al.*, 1986, p.145)

Such a view gives strong support to the concept of normalisation as developed by Wolfensberger and others (Wolfensberger, 1972, 1980; Campaign for Mentally Handicapped People, 1981). While focusing on the physical environment, it stresses the need to allow people who are devalued by society to regain control over their lives.

Of course, elderly people may need the support of staff to enable them to maximise their potential. However, it should be recognised that such relationships are not one-sided. It is not a case of 'them and us', independence or dependence, but interdependency. While it is important for us to redress the institutional environment in favour of the resident/patient, we need to remember that institutions are also work environments for staff, and often it is the separation of living and working environments which provides the greatest barrier to attempts to bring about change. In this way working practices should not start from the premise of 'what is the most efficient use of my time?' but 'how can I help this individual to achieve a satisfactory lifestyle in his or her terms?' Such views demand not only adequate resources in terms of staffing and facilities, but also a change in attitudes among staff, and society at large, as to how we value old people who are coming to the end of their lives.

Given this range of issues, how do we bring about change in institutional settings? In drawing on the findings of the National Consumer Study, Willcocks *et al.* (1982, 1986) made a series of recommendations concerning the future of residential environments for old people, which focused on a change from public living in communal space to private living in personal space. While these recommendations were given shape in the form of a new building design based on 'residential flatlets' plus supportive services (see Figure 15.1), the underlying conditions for a change in institutional practice were deemed of more fundamental importance. They included the following (Peace *et al.*, 1982, p. 48):

- The transformation of spatial arrangements in the home.
- The introduction of practical measures to ensure the right kind of organisational support for this new lifestyle — i.e. institutional change through staff training programmes.
- A positive shift in the relationship between the residential home and the community at large.

Thus, the authors illustrate how change can only be brought about by a total reappraisal of all facets of institutional life, and suggest that in this way you can 'break down the walls of the institution' so that it can be seen as a part of community care; thus revaluing institutional provision.

The views espoused above have become more pertinent in recent years with the growth of private residential care and the enactment of the *Registered Homes Act 1984* and the *Residential Care Homes Regulations 1984*. While the mandatory aspects of legislation focus attention on the physical environment (the fit building), staffing (the fit persons) and standards such as fire safety, sanitation, medication and record-keeping, the accompanying Code of Practice, *Home Life*, addresses itself not only to these issues, but also to the principles of care — its philosophy and practice (Centre for Policy on Ageing, 1984). The following introduction of these principles reaffirms the importance of how we value the individual:

> . . . underlying all the recommendations and requirements set out in this Code is a conviction that those who live in residential care should do so with dignity;

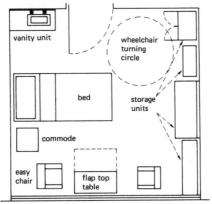

sketch layout of resident's living-room (15 m² approx.)

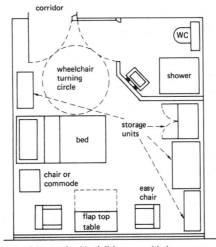

sketch layout of resident's living-room with shower room
and WC en suite (18 m² approx.)

Figure 15.1 Residential flatlet. Support services also provided in the form of:

- Sanitary services such as a vanity unit would form an integral part of the flatlet, or be located adjacent to it, as would the shower plus WC. Baths would be provided separately.
- Two levels of catering: (1) centrally prepared and served meals for those who chose to be served; (2) kitchenettes for those who wish to help themselves.
- At least one large lounge, possibly incorporating part of the entrance hall, as an alternative meeting-place.

Source: Willcocks *et al.* (1986, pp. 150–151)

that they should have the respect of those who support them; should live with
no reduction of their rights as citizens (except where the law so prescribes), and
should be entitled to live as full and active a life as their physical and mental
condition will allow.

(Centre for Policy on Ageing, 1984, p. 15)

The Code reinforces the importance of residents' rights and stresses the
value attached to the maintenance of personal dignity, access to private
space, choice, autonomy, and responsible risk-taking. If we wish to promote
a more enlightened institutional environment for old people, then just how
far registering authorities use the Code as a tool for establishing good
practice will be crucial. If our energies become exhausted in trying solely to
maintain the more material standards, then we shall have failed. If this
happens, then, once again, we shall find ourselves asking not how we
promote the 'right' institutional environment, but whether we can, and
whether we should.

HOW FAR CAN WE ACHIEVE CHANGE WITHIN INSTITUTIONS?

Very few people seem to realise that valued people are virtually never
segregated from society against their will and that one will only see such
segregation when people are devalued.

(Wolfensberger, 1980, p. 77)

On reading this comment by Wolfensberger, some may say that this does not
apply to old people living in institutional settings; that many have chosen to
move into a care setting and can exercise a level of control over their lives.
Yet, to date, research concerning both public and private residential
provision would suggest that there is some truth here; that choice over
residential living in late life may be constrained, and that in some cases a
form of subtle coercion exists on the part of professionals and family alike
which makes institutional care the only solution to the needs of some frail
elderly people (Willcocks *et al.*, 1982; Weaver *et al.*, 1985). Of course, such
coercion commonly is not deliberate, but, as we have seen, a combination of
factors — the increase in the numbers of the 'old' old; the growing pressure
on community resources; changes in family structure and roles; and the
promotion of private care — are all contributing to the likelihood that more
old people will experience some form of institutional living in later life.

If the demand for institutional care increases, then we might expect a call
from consumers for a better quality of environment more suited to their
needs. Yet, while this may be the case for the healthy, middle-class, elderly
who actively seek alternative living environments, it may not be the case for
those more passive consumers — predominantly frail older women with
restricted means — for whom choice is limited. As a consequence, the

responsibility for seeking to change current practice within institutional settings lies not only with those who work with old people, but also with the wider community, the potential consumers of the future.

But is such change possible? At present it appears that a number of interrelated factors may actively work against such progress. First, as we have seen, there is the strength of the institution, the bureaucratic pull which makes it easier to provide a service geared to the homogeneous needs of a homogeneous group. Can this be overcome? Second, there is the lack of co-ordination and communication between those who provide services for the frail elderly; the division between public, private and voluntary sectors, between housing, health and social services. Such fragmentation reflects the unique historical development of different professional groupings who now have a common concern in providing alternative living environments for old people, but have yet to develop a common framework through which to channel the important contribution that each has to make. Nowhere is this disjunction exposed more blatantly than within the current debate over the dual registration of residential and nursing homes, where a battle for supremacy between nursing and residential models of care could completely cloud the more fundamental concern of providing a client-centred service. Thus, both service systems and institutional norms marginalise the individual, a situation which is made worse by the commonly held negative attitude towards old age. Such attitudes are reflected not only in the treatment of the old, but also in the low status afforded to those who work with elderly people, and the limited resources available to them.

Finally, within institutional settings the devalued status of old people is compounded further by the fact that a majority of residents/patients die within these environments. Given that death is considered taboo within our society, it is hardly surprising that this important fact of institutional life often goes unnoted, internalised within our negative image of the setting. As a consequence, when we talk about promoting change within institutions, it is common to emphasis the 'positive' aspects of institutional life — companionship, rehabilitation, activity, self-maintenance — which may raise the morale of both staff and residents/patients. Yet, while recognising the importance of these factors, I would argue that as long as we deny the presence of death within the institution, we shall also fail to create an environment that encompasses all aspects of institutional life. Nowhere is this more clearly demonstrated than in the contrast that exists between the highly respected personalised care provided by the hospice movement (see Taylor, 1983) and the negative image which still surrounds the residential home, the nursing home, the geriatric ward.

In conclusion, we must acknowledge that at a time when institutional living for frail elderly people at the end of their lives may be increasing, there are also a number of forces which appear to actively work against radical change in such settings. If such obstacles are to be overcome, then progress needs to occur at several levels. We have already seen that much can be done to improve the physical environments and care practices within institutions. However, in order to create settings where old people are valued, we still have to find ways of replacing the dependent status commonly attached to elderly residents/patients, and its connotation of helplessness, with attitudes that recognise the potential for interdependence and reciprocity between residents/patients, staff and relatives: an interdependence not just at the level of activity, but also with respect to past experience and life history. In this way we may achieve the ultimate goal where institutional care is seen as another part of community care; without such a reappraisal it may prove impossible to promote the 'right' institutional environment.

REFERENCES

Booth, T. (1985). *Home Truths: Old People's Homes and the Outcome of Care*. Gower Press, Aldershot
Campaign for Mentally Handicapped People (1981). *The Principle of Normalisation: A Foundation for Effective Services*. Campaign for Mentally Handicapped People, London
Centre for Policy on Ageing (1984). *Home Life: A Code of Practice for Residential Care* (Report of a Working Party Sponsored by the DHSS and convened by the Centre for Policy on Ageing under the Chairmanship of Kina, Lady Avebury). Centre for Policy on Ageing, London
Department of Health and Social Security and Welsh Office (1962). *Local Authority Building Note No. 2: Residential Accommodation for Elderly People*. HMSO, London
Department of Health and Social Security and Welsh Office (1973). *Local Authority Building Note No. 2: Residential Accommodation for Elderly People*. HMSO, London
Fengler, A., Kellaher, L.A. and Peace, S. M. (1985). *The Meaning of Home for Elderly Widowed Homeowners: Consequences for the Decision to Move or to Homeshare*. Working Paper, Centre for Environmental and Social Studies in Ageing, Polytechnic of North London
Goffman, I. (1961). *Asylums*. Doubleday Anchor, New York
Golant, S. (1982). Individual differences underlying the dwelling satisfaction of the elderly. *J. Social Issues*, **38**, 121
Howell, S. (1983). The meaning of place in old age. In Rowles, G. and Ohta, R. (Eds.), *Ageing and Milieu: Environmental Perspectives on Growing Old*, pp. 97–107. Academic Press, New York
Jones, K. and Fowles, A. J. (1984). *Ideas on Institutions: Analysing the Literature on Long-term Care and Custody*. Routledge and Kegan Paul, London
Kastenbaum, R. (1983). Can the clinical milieu be therapeutic? In Rowles, G.D. and Ohta, R. J. (Eds.), *Ageing and Milieu: Environmental Perspectives on Growing Old*, pp. 3–16. Academic Press, New York
King, R. D., Raynes, N. V. and Tizard, J. (1971). *Patterns of Residential Care*. Routledge and Kegan Paul, London
Lawton, M. P. (1980). *Environment and Ageing*. Brooks/Cole, Monterey

Lawton, M. P. (1983). Environment and other determinants of well-being in older people. *Gerontologist*, **23** (4), 349

Lawton, M. P. and Nahemow, L. (1973). Ecology and the ageing process. In Eisdorfer, C. and Lawton, M. P. (Eds.), *The Psychology of Adult Development and Ageing*. American Psychological Association, Washington D.C.

Leibowitz, B. (1978). Implications of community housing for planning and policy. *Gerontologist*, **2** (18), 140

Means, R. and Smith, R. (1983). From public assistance institutions to 'Sunshine Hotels': changing State perceptions about residential care for elderly people, 1939–48. *Ageing and Society*, **3**, 157

National Assistance Act (1948). HMSO, London

O'Bryant, S. L. (1983). The subjective value of 'home' to older homeowners. *J. Housing Elderly*, **1** (1), 29

Office of Population Censuses and Surveys (1983). *Persons of Pensionable Age, Great Britain* (Census 1981). HMSO, London

Peace, S. M. (1986a). Residential accommodation for dependent elderly people in Britain: the relationship between spatial structure and individual lifestyle. Paper presented at the *Franco-British Symposium on the Geography of Ageing in Britain and France, Age Concern Institute of Gerontology, King's College, London, July 1986*

Peace, S. M. (1986b). The design of residential homes: an historical perspective. In Judge, K. and Sinclair, I. (Eds.), *Residential Care for Elderly People*, pp. 139–150. HMSO, London

Peace, S. M. and Harding, S. D. (1980). *An Evaluation of Group Living in Residential Homes for the Elderly in the London Borough of Haringey*. Research Report No. 2., Survey Research Unit, Polytechnic of North London

Peace, S. M., Kellaher, L. A. and Willcocks, D. M. (1982). *A Balanced Life. A Consumer Study of Residential Life in 100 Local Authority Old People's Homes*. Research Report No. 14, Survey Research Unit, Polytechnic of North London

Peace, S. M., with Nusberg, C. (1984). *Shared Living: A Viable Alternative for the Elderly*. International Federation on Ageing, Washington, D.C.

Raynes, N. V., Pratt, M. W. and Roses, S. (1979). *Organisational Structure and the Care of the Mentally Retarded*. Croom Helm, London

Registered Homes Act (1984). HMSO, London

Residential Care Homes Regulations (1984). No. 1345. HMSO, London

Rowles, G. (1983). Place and personal identity in old age: observations from Appalachia. *J. Envir. Psychol.*, **3**, 299

Sixsmith, A. (1986). Independence and home in later life. In Phillipson, C., Bernard, M. and Strang, P. (Eds.), *Dependency and Interdependency in Old Age: Theoretical Perspectives and Policy Alternatives*. Croom Helm, London

Swenarton, M. (1981). *Homes Fit For Heroes: The Politics and Architecture of Early State Housing in Britain*. Heinemann Educational, London

Taylor, H. (1983). *The Hospice Movement in Britain: Its Role and Its Future*. Report No. 2, Centre for Policy on Ageing, London

Tinker, A. (1984). *The Elderly in Modern Society*, 2nd edn. Longman, London

Townsend, P. (1962). *The Last Refuge*. Routledge and Kegan Paul, London

Townsend, J. and Kimbell, A. (1975). Caring regimes in elderly persons' homes. *Hlth Soc. Serv. J.*, 11 October, 2286

Weaver, T., Willcocks, D. and Kellaher, L. (1985). *The Business of Care: A Study of Private Residential Homes for Older People*. Research Report No. 1, Centre for Environmental and Social Studies in Ageing, Polytechnic of North London

Wheeler, R. (1985). *Don't Move: We've Got you Covered. A Study of the Anchor Housing Trust Staying Put Scheme*. Institute of Housing, London

Willcocks, D. M., Peace, S. M. and Kellaher, L. A. (1986). *Private Lives in Public Places: A Research-based Critique of Residential Life in Local Authority Old People's Homes*. Tavistock, London

Willcocks, D. M., Peace, S. M. and Kellaher, L. A., with Ring, A. J. (1982). *The Residential Life of Old People: A Study of 100 Local Authority Homes*, Vol. 1. Research Report No. 12, Survey Research Unit, Polytechnic of North London

Wing, J. K. and Brown, G. W. (1970). *Institutionalisation and Schizophrenia*. Cambridge University Press, Cambridge

Wolfensberger, W. (1972). *The Principle of Normalization in Human Services*. National Institute on Mental Retardation, Toronto

Wolfensberger, W. (1980). The definition of normalization: update, problems, disagreements and misunderstandings. In Flynn, R. J. and Nitson, K. E. (Eds.), *Normalization, Social Integration and Community Services*, pp. 71–116. University Park Press, Baltimore

16

Living Environments for the Elderly. 3: The Mixed Economy in Long-term Care

William Laing

INTRODUCTION

One of the most far-reaching and least remarked upon changes in the Welfare State in recent years has been the shift from public to private provision of long-term residential and nursing care of elderly people. In 1975 an estimated 16 per cent of elderly people in long-term care in England lived in private nursing and residential homes. By the end of 1985 this proportion had risen to 37 per cent (Table 16.1; Figure 16.1). If, as seems likely, local

Table 16.1 Elderly people in long-term care, 1975–1985/86 (1000s)

	1975	1985/86
Private nursing homes	13	29 (Dec. 1985)
Private residential homes	19	79 (Mar. 1986)
Total private sector	32 (16%)	108 (37%)
Voluntary nursing homes	4	4
Voluntary residential homes	22	26
Total voluntary sector	26 (13%)	30 (10%)
Local Authority homes	95	102
NHS long-stay geriatric patients	36	31
NHS elderly severely mentally ill	16	20
Total public sector	147 (72%)	153 (53%)
All sectors	205	291

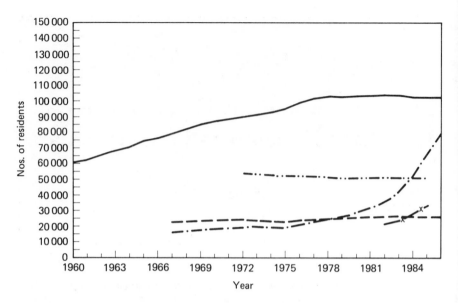

Figure 16.1 Residents aged 65 and over by type of institution, England, 1960–86.
—, Local authority; —·—, private residential homes; – – – , voluntary residential
homes; —×—×, nursing homes; —··—··, NHS long-stay. Sources: DHSS Residential Accommodation Statistics for local authority provided and registered residential
accommodation, with estimates for March 1986 based on local authority
registrations. SBH 212 returns for nursing homes, adjusted for bed occupancy and
estimated for 1985 on the basis of health authority registrations (includes places not
specified as designated for non-elderly client groups)

authority and voluntary provision remain at a standstill and National Health
Service geriatric departments continue their withdrawal from long-
term care (mitigated to some extent by an increase in psychogeriatric
provision), the private sector will have to provide all the volume growth
necessary to keep pace with demographic change. Its share of the 'mixed
economy' may thus reach 50 per cent by the turn of the century. What does
this change mean for those elderly people who spend the last months or
years of their lives in some form of communal establishment? And what are
the prospects for the future?

THE DEMAND FOR ACCOMMODATION

Only an estimated 4 per cent of British people over 65 years of age live in
communal establishments offering personal or nursing care, although the
percentage rises very rapidly with increasing age. Just how rapidly is
illustrated in Figure 16.2, which relates to residential care only (that is, local
authority, private and voluntary residential homes combined, for elderly

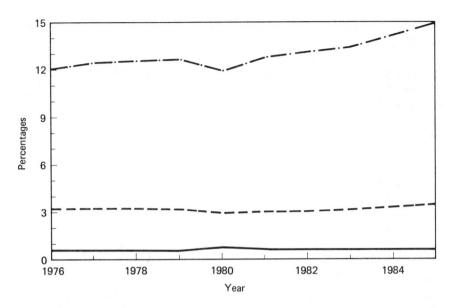

Figure 16.2 Percentage of population resident in local authority, private and voluntary residential homes for elderly and physically handicapped people by age group, England, 1976–85. —, 65–74; – – – , 75–84; —·—, 85+. Source: DHSS Residential Accommodation Statistics

and physically disabled people). According to local authority returns to the Department of Health and Social Security (DHSS), about 15 per cent of the English population aged 85 years and over live in these establishments. When hospital and nursing home residents are added in, the proportion rises to about 20 per cent.

The principal demographic change facing Britain in the 1980s is the growth of the 'old old' population, which is expected to continue beyond the end of the century and to fuel the demand for long-term care. Because there are so many more very old people in the population, residential homes have become dominated by this client group — a trend which has given rise to concern, since many old people's homes now have to cater for a mix of clientele for which they were never intended, including frequently high proportions of mentally confused people. Inevitably, this has had a detrimental impact on living environments, particularly in local authority homes, which tend to cater for more dependent individuals (Association of Directors of Social Services, 1985).

It is worth noting, however, that the ageing of residential home populations is *not* a consequence of successful community care policies keeping younger people in their own homes, whatever the wishful thinking of government or directors of social services. In so far as the DHSS residential accommodation statistics are reliable (and those for 1981 are broadly

validated by independent census data), the past decade has seen no
significant reduction in the probability of either younger (under 65 years)
and 'young old' (65–74 years) individuals living in a residential home. For
age groups over 75 years, and particularly for those over 85 years, the
probability of living in a residential home remained fairly constant until the
early 1980s, since when it has significantly increased, at least partly as a
consequence of the availability of supplementary benefits funding for
private residential care (Figure 16.2).

The stark fact is that investment in local authority sheltered housing and
community services for elderly people during the last decade has had no
discernible impact on the volume of residential care required.

The conclusion to be drawn is that, in the absence of new and more
effectively supportive models of sheltered housing and community care
(about which, more later), the number of people living in institutional
settings will grow inexorably with the ageing population. On the basis of
constant age-specific rates of occupation, the number of residents in
communal establishments in England can be projected to increase from
291 000 in 1986 to 358 000 by the turn of the century. And on present trends,
all of this increase will be located in the private sector (Figure 16.3).

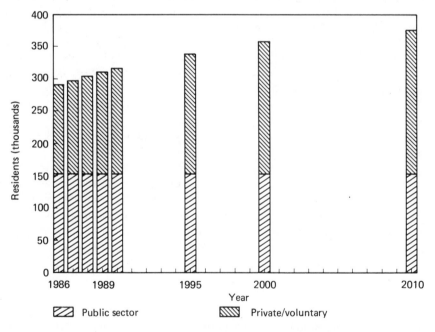

Figure 16.3 Projected residents aged 65 years and over in hospitals, nursing homes
and residential homes, England, 1986–2010. Note: Derived by application of 1986
age-specific rates of occupation to Office of Population Censuses and Surveys
population projections assuming static public sector provision

LIVING ENVIRONMENTS

Despite often dedicated personal and nursing attention, it remains a fact that most elderly people in long-term care live in drab and unappealing environments in which it is difficult to maintain privacy, dignity and such autonomy as physical and mental frailty allows. Throughout the public, private and voluntary sectors, with some notable exceptions, there is a prevailing poverty of imagination which, alongside frequently tightly restrained resources, deprives elderly people of attractive and supportive living conditions and the sort of amenities that most residents would previously have taken for granted. Care of elderly people is one of the very last service sectors to respond to the post-war tide of consumerism which has transformed the standard of amenity and service demanded elsewhere.

Regarding long-term care in National Health Service hospitals, the 1985/6 report of the Health Advisory Service (1986) makes depressing reading. It notes: ' . . . the brazen neglect of years gone by has been replaced by a pattern of care which is hygienic but still predominantly institutional'. Care received in the private sector is certainly more homely, because of both smaller-scale units and the absence of a medical ethos, while such independent evaluation as has been carried out (for example, Day and Klein, 1985) indicates that alarmist reports of unacceptably low quality of care in profit-making homes (for example, National Union of Public Employees, 1986) relate to only a small minority of establishments. But typical standards of amenity nevertheless remain poor. The results of a survey of 158 private and voluntary residential homes carried out in early 1985 provide an illustration of some measurable indicators of amenity such as single-room occupation and private bathrooms. Only about half of the residents occupied a single room at that time, and fewer than 10 per cent had their own bathroom (Tables 16.2, 16.3). *Home Life*, the code of practice for residential homes, recommends single rooms where possible (Centre for Policy on

Table 16.2 Room occupancy (%). Source: Office of Health Economics Survey of 158 residential and nursing homes, end 1984

	Nursing homes		Residential homes		
Occupancy	*Private*	*Voluntary*	*Private*	*Voluntary*	*All homes*
Single	39	72	52	57	51
Double	33	14	31	21	29
Multiple	28	14	17	21	20
All occupancies	100	100	100	100	100

Table 16.3 En suite bathrooms by charge level. Source: Office of Health Economics Survey of 158 private and voluntary residential and nursing homes, end 1984

Charges (£/week)	% with en suite bathroom
250+	48
200–	30
180–	15
160–	17
140–	14
120–	9
100–	7
80–	4
under 60	3
All charges	9

Ageing, 1984) and local authorities are now implementing this, but there is no such recommendation in the National Association of Health Authorities' corresponding guidelines for nursing homes (1985).

THE PRIVATE SECTOR — WILL IT EXTEND CHOICE?

Because of its growing importance in supply and innovation, and because relatively little has been written about it, the following discussion of the mixed economy of welfare is concerned principally with *private*-sector activity, and whether and how it can offer increased access to a range of different forms of care about which consumers and their agents can make informed choices in the light of costs.

Broadly, two sets of factors, regulatory and market-related, will have a bearing on prospects for improving living environments of elderly people opting for long-term care in the private sector.

Regulatory Factors

The fundamental presumption of the 1984 *Registered Homes Act* is that neither the exercise of individual choice nor self-regulation by suppliers is sufficient to protect vulnerable consumers from exploitation. This proposition is accepted across most of the political spectrum. The first two years of operation of the *Act* have seen substantial progress towards its principal objectives of eradicating that small minority of homes where standards of care are unacceptably low and excluding operators unfit to run homes. These are, of course, fairly minimal objectives. Over and above that, there is the question of whether the style and nature of local and health authority regulation, and the precedents set by the Homes Tribunals, act to increase or restrict such choice as consumers and their agents are able to exercise.

One potentially major concern, which has received little attention, is the threat to traditional 'cottage industry' owner-managers with residential homes of less than 20 places. This arises principally from the minimum staffing recommendations of *Home Life*. To the extent that local authorities decide rigorously to implement them, residential homes below about 20 places could be placed at a serious cost disadvantage. A (presumably unwanted) side-effect would be to raise significant barriers to entry for traditional prospective home-owners with limited capital resources. Al- though there is as yet no clear evidence of any such barriers developing in the first two years of the *Act*'s operation, it is something that should be monitored closely. Potential consequences include an increase in the number of employed home managers, a loss of one of the few opportunities for self-employment among women in middle life, and a reduction in choice for consumers who value the special quality of personal commitment that is characteristic of owner-managed homes.

Local authority regulation may also reduce choice at the opposite end of the range. The almost universal view in social service departments is that personal care is best delivered in small homely units, and this has led many authorities to impose a size limit on any home seeking registration. In some counties this is as low as 25 places.

The alternative view, articulated by some corporate operators, is that many elderly people — particularly those with substantial res- ources — would prefer the sort of facilities that can only be economically provided in a larger establishment. Social service departments, they argue, are using regulatory processes to impose a very restricted view of the living environments that elderly people want in residential care, one that arises from dealing with a particular range of clientele in their own Part III homes. Without passing judgement on the merits of either view, this is clearly an issue worthy of debate. It may also have an important bearing on the pace and direction of innovation within the private sector, since many commercial 'continuing care community' concepts involve fairly large (50 beds or more) dual-registration establishments whose style of operation is closer to that of a hotel than that of a traditional old persons' home.

A more unambiguously positive effect of the degree of regulation to which the residential and nursing homes are now subject is the encouragement of new-build homes. This is not an intended effect, but arises coincidently from the high cost of meeting more rigorous requirements in converted property. It has meant that the new-build cost is now very close to the cost of rehabilitation. Up to very recently, virtually all private nursing and residen- tial homes were in converted property. For the first time, some developers are now building new. Though new-build will not be to everyone's taste, its emergence in the private sector represents a significant extension of choice, with a number of (potential) advantages in design, staffing efficiency and energy costs.

Local authority planning departments will also have a significant impact on the development of continuing care communities offering sheltered housing, and residential and nursing care on the same site. Only a handful of these schemes exists at present, principally in the voluntary sector, although it is in the private sector that interest in developing new projects is at its greatest. Suitable sites are not easy to find, and the attitudes adopted by local authority planners will be a key determinant of the pace at which this form of social experimentation can take place.

The most powerful influence exercised by the public sector over living environments in private residential and nursing homes, however, is that directly affecting recipients of supplementary benefits (SB). Since April 1985, SB limits have been set at levels which are barely adequate to meet the costs of modest establishments in most areas. National SB limits were an emergency measure to curb the spiralling cost to the DHSS of supporting elderly people in private and voluntary homes. But though they effectively reduced the unit cost of care, the number of individuals receiving support in Britain continued to escalate, from 42 500 in December 1984 to an estimated 90 000 in February 1986, in the absence of need assessment or any control on eligibility other than a means test. Though work conducted by the Social Policy Research Unit at the University of York suggests that all but a small minority of SB-funded residents of residential care homes 'need' to be there on ordinary local authority criteria, there is nevertheless concern that many individuals are not aware of all the alternatives and may be steered into an inappropriate living environment.

In 1987, however, the opportunity exists to institute a more rational system of income support which does not discriminate against community care. The first shot in what is likely to be a hard fought debate came with the publication of the DHSS/Local Authority Association's Second Joint Working Party on Supplementary Benefit and Residential Care (DHSS, 1987). One of its key recommendations was that the money then spent on SB support should be transferred over to the control of local authorities. Such a transfer would probably be the most effective means of controlling total expenditure, but at the cost of limiting the choice that is implicit in SB funding, albeit imperfectly exercised by highly vulnerable consumers. These issues will be confronted once again by the high-powered Griffiths working group on community care, set up after the highly critical Audit Commission report (Audit Commission, 1986) and due to report by the end of 1987. Funding of institutional and community care are inextricably interrelated and one of the principal challenges faced by Griffiths is to create a structure in which appropriate incentives exist in that grey area where choice between institutional and community care is finely balanced. The linchpin of any new funding structure which retains supplementary benefits is likely to be need assessment. This offers the vital control mechanism which can allow a voucher system of funding, which is in essence what supplementary benefit support represents, to a range of community care services for a wider clientele without unacceptable cost consequences, and for financial support to be varied in a coherent manner according to individual need. For example, benefit for home care may be restricted to those who would otherwise be eligible for residential or nursing home support, in a manner analogous to experiments set up in the 1970s within Kent's Department of Social Services.

An important opportunity exists for greatly rationalising the system of support for people with limited financial resources of their own. With the right decisions, substantial progress may be made, within the cost constraints under which government inevitably operates, in extending real choices available to frail and dependent elderly people seeking more appropriate and supportive living environments.

Market Factors

Principally, the growth of the private sector over the last few years has represented more of the same thing — that is, 'cottage industry' proprietors setting up homes along traditional lines to deal with a known demand. The engine of growth has been the ageing population, greatly assisted by the availability of supplementary benefits.

But it should be emphasised that the majority of private home residents pay their fees out of their own, or their families', pockets. At the top end of the privately financed market, some of the cottage industry proprietors and newly emergent corporate operators are breaking new ground in a limited way by offering a higher standard of amenity than has been available hitherto — for example, single rooms with *en suite* bathrooms, albeit with fairly small room sizes.

Much more radical and potentially more significant private sector innovation is now taking place at the interface between sheltered housing and residential and nursing care. Typically, new packages of accommodation and care being offered require substantial capital investment and entail a higher degree of risk for providers. They are, therefore, outside the range of the traditional cottage industry operator.

INNOVATION: FROM SHELTERED HOUSING TO 'LIFE CARE' COMMUNITIES

Until very recently, sheltered housing in Britain was almost entirely the preserve of local authorities and housing associations. Between them they provided 468 000 out of the 470 000 units estimated to exist in 1980. In 1977 McCarthy and Stone became the first company to offer flats for sale exclusively to elderly people, and by 1985, 31 000 units had been completed or were in the course of construction. The estimated potential market is between 250 000 and 400 000 units (Baker and Parry, 1986).

Sheltered housing units for sale, as originally conceived by McCarthy and Stone, were small, town-centre, self-contained flats with an emergency alarm system, normally a resident warden and communal facilities, including a laundry room, a common room and a bedroom for visiting guests. According to Baker and Parry, such developments changed little between 1977 and 1983.

One of the criticisms of much sheltered housing for sale has been that units have not been designed to meet the needs of elderly people as they grow older and more frail. Often leases require residents to move if they become dependent. Few developments incorporate design features to facilitate home care for frail elderly people (e.g. wide doorways, level handles, high-level sockets), and many are built on more than one storey without a lift. Some commentators maintain that the private sector is now in the process of repeating the mistakes of public-sector sheltered housing developments a decade or more ago. It is failing to design living environments in which elderly people who grow frail and dependent can be supported in the community without the necessity of entering residential or nursing care.

In the last few years, however, the sheltered housing market has become segmented. As part of the process of segmentation, a number of innovative models have been developed which could add significantly to choice, at least among affluent elderly people, to whom they are principally being marketed. Expanded packages of services and facilities are being offered in order to achieve a higher premium on sale prices or service charges. These may include domestic cleaning, meals, laundry, shopping services, leisure facilities and domiciliary services including an element of personal care. At their most extensive, services may include residential and nursing care, though only a handful of such developments exist as yet.

The 'life care' or 'continuing care community' concept is the most radically innovative model. It may also prove the most difficult to sell. It not only seeks to serve a clientele ranging (ultimately) from recently retired couples to frail and dependent widows and widowers, but also aims to offer an assurance of permanent care for those who become too dependent to look after themselves. 'Life care' has much in common with long-established voluntary sector communities in Britain, but the inspiration for private-sector developments has to date come principally from American models.

The appeal of 'life care' communities, however, may be limited for two reasons. The first relates to the nature of the product. Some people, especially younger retired, may find the existence of long-term nursing care on the same site unattractive, suggesting, as it does, the inevitability of physical and mental decline. (Why not a mortuary to complete the chain?)

The second reason is the absence of sound actuarial data, which makes insurance cover against the risk of needing long-term nursing care either unavailable or prohibitively expensive. This is one of a number of examples of market failure in this new sector of corporate activity.

Mixed client developments represent a somewhat less ambitious model than full-blown 'life care'. Here the sheltered housing and residential/nursing care activities are financially self-contained. This avoids the insurance problem. At the same time, the scale of development allows a range of common services to be offered. There is also scope for some trading activities — for example, the residential/nursing home may provide meals and emergency on-call services for the adjacent sheltered housing development. A number of such developments are in the pipeline, and they are likely to become increasingly common, since they make an attractive development package for builders and residential/nursing home operators.

Very sheltered housing, as developed by Retirement Security Ltd, is worthy of special mention, since it represents the only coherent model of sheltered housing which might plausibly provide a wholly non-institutional substitute for residential and even some nursing home care. Retirement Security is a private company headed by Bob Bessell, who, while Director of Social Services at Warwickshire, noted the failure of conventional public-sector sheltered housing to prevent entry into residential care. Very sheltered housing offers a wider than usual package of support services, including domiciliary help and a restaurant. It provides a higher level of warden service than most sheltered housing, and wardens' job descriptions emphasise supporting the independence of residents rather than simply providing emergency cover. Service charges are higher than average, but are frequently covered by social security benefits. If very sheltered housing can prove over time that it offers a substitute for residential care, then the quality of life benefits would be substantial, since the overwhelming majority of people express a preference to stay in their own homes, given adequate support (Tinker, 1984).

THE CHALLENGE OF FINANCING PROVISION

With the possible exception of very sheltered housing, all innovative activity in private-sector care of elderly people is aimed at satisfying the preferences and needs of the most wealthy 5 per cent of the population, most of whom live in the south-east. The challenge facing providers of private care now is to bring innovative models and potential for better living environments within the reach of the bulk of the elderly population. The principal source of private funding that will have to be tapped is the capital tied up in elderly owner-occupiers' present homes.

At the beginning of the nineteenth century, when people now entering sheltered housing and residential/nursing care were born, only 8 per cent of housing was owner-occupied. Today some 50 per cent of householders over retirement age are owner-occupiers. For single adult households over the age of 60 (mainly elderly widows — the principal clientele for sheltered housing and residential/nursing care), the 1982 General Household Survey shows 38 per cent owner-occupation, all but 2 per cent without a mortgage. Thus, a large — and rising — proportion of people have a more or less substantial capital asset at their disposal, which could be used to fund different forms of care and accommodation.

For those who are capable of looking after themselves, there is now a variety of methods of releasing capital from owner-occupied property to fund the creation of more appropriate and supportive living environments. Interest-only loans can be obtained for improvements to an existing home, or part of a large house can be retained and the remainder sold to finance conversion and improvement. 'Home for life' and similar private funding schemes allow elderly people to buy sheltered housing below cost, in return for reversion of the property on death to the financing organisation. Thus, within the constraints of the existing distribution of wealth — and individuals' ability to make use of it — the market has responded with mechanisms for enhancing living environments for this less dependent client group. Applying the Nationwide Building Society's (1986) statistics on house price distribution, new sheltered housing or its equivalent is potentially within the reach of about half to three-quarters of present owner-occupiers.

For more dependent clientele, however, the market has as yet failed to provide efficient mechanisms for translating owner-occupiers' capital into funding of long-term residential or nursing care.

Many elderly people pay residential or nursing home fees by selling their previous homes. The money raised may be invested to bear interest or an annuity may be purchased. But each method is financially inefficient, since the low interest paid to home residents is being used, partly, to finance high-interest borrowings of home-owners. To avoid this would require direct equity participation by the resident in the home. No private-sector organisation has yet resolved the complex legal and financial problems involved, although one company, Trustcare plc, launched a new venture in 1986 which may, in time, offer a form of owner-occupation to residential/nursing home clientele. Their proposals involve vesting the freehold of a communal establishment in a trust, which, in turn, employs a management company to provide hotel and care services. With the trust protecting the residents' interests, this provides the vitally important guarantee that a resident's investment will not be compromised by arbitrary changes in the price and content of these services.

Another gap in the supply side of the market — and one which substantially reduces consumer choice and ability to fund high-quality care — relates to the lack of insurance and financial services, interest in addressing the needs of individuals entering residential or nursing homes. There are, for example, no insurance policies or pension plans designed specifically for younger people to cover themselves against the risk of future admission to long-term care. One reason is the perceived lack of demand for such insurance. But another reason may simply be the absence of any reliable actuarial data on risk of admission and length of stay.

Much more important, for those older individuals on the point of entering long-term care, is the absence of affordable financial products offering security that care will be funded till death.

At present, such products are limited to index-linked annuity plans. But their costs put them beyond the means of most people. For example, at rates ruling in 1986, an 80-year-old woman would typically pay £65 000–£97 500 in order to receive £200–£300 per week to cover good-quality nursing care till death. Probably less than 5 per cent of individuals entering care have capital of that magnitude. However, evidence is emerging from a number of surveys of residential and nursing homes (for example, Bartlett and Challis, 1986) which suggests that the expectation of life of individuals entering long-term care is considerably less than that of individuals of the same age within the general population. General life tables indicate that the 80-year-old woman quoted above has a life expectation in excess of 7 years, and the cost of her annuity would be based on this. But in reality the expectation of life of an individual entering long-term care is probably much less. The problem is that there are no life tables relating to this subpopulation of particularly frail and dependent individuals. If there were, it is quite possible the cost of annuities could be halved. The importance of this is that it would bring lifetime funding of long-term care within the means of the owner of a typical semidetached house.

Of course, funding of long-term care with accumulated capital has its corollary that family members will not receive the inheritance they might otherwise have looked forward to. For this reason, there may be consider-able family resistance to this avenue for improving living environments for elderly people. It is a conflict of conscience and interest that is likely to become increasingly common as a new, more demanding generation of elderly people starts entering care and as awareness percolates through society that the zero-price option of long-term care within the National Health Service is no longer available.

REFERENCES

Association of Directors of Social Services (1985). *Who Goes Where?* Association of Directors of Social Services
Audit Commission (1986). *Making a Reality of Community Care.* HMSO, London

Baker, S. and Parry, M. J. (1986). *Housing for Sale to the Elderly: Third Report.* Housing Research Foundation, London

Bartlett, H. and Challis, L. (1986). Private Nursing Homes for the Elderly: Working Paper 3. Centre for the Analysis of Social Policy, University of Bath

Centre for Policy on Ageing (1984). *Home Life: A Code of Practice for Residential Care.* Centre for Policy on Ageing, London

Day, P. and Klein, R. (1985). Maintaining standards in the independent sector of health care. *Br. Med. J.*, **290**, 1020

Department of Health and Social Security (1987). *Public Support for Residential Care: Report of a Joint Central and Local Government Working Party*

Health Advisory Service (1986). *Annual Report* of the Health Advisory Service, 1985/86

National Association of Health Authorities (1985). *Registration and Inspection of Nursing Homes: A Handbook for Health Authorities.* National Association of Health Authorities in England and Wales, Birmingham

National Union of Public Employees (1986). *Time for Justice: NUPE's Report on Care of the Elderly.* NUPE, London

Nationwide Building Society (1986). Data on prices of houses purchased with a Nationwide mortage, 1st quarter 1986

Tinker, A. (1984). *Staying at Home: Helping Elderly People.* HMSO, London

17
Economic Resources and Ageing

Alan Maynard

INTRODUCTION

Any discussion of the care of the elderly seems inevitably to add to the demands for greater funding. The purpose of this chapter is to examine briefly these demands at the macro and micro levels.

At the macro level of the global funding of the heterogeneous collection of public and private caring activities, it seems that the additional resource demands may be modest. However, this conclusion is tentative and is made on the basis of incomplete economic and epidemiological knowledge. The issues of system resource demands and epidemiological knowledge are explored in the next section.

Any discussion of the micro economics of caring policies for the elderly brings out the chaotic nature of financing and provision, arising from the compartmentalisation of the market and the existence of perverse incentives, which, in the absence of a patient advocate who is the system's budget holder, results in inefficient use of resources and a failure to care for the elderly in a cost-effective manner. It is these issues which form the substance of the second section of this chapter.

RESOURCE REQUIREMENTS AND THE EPIDEMIOLOGY OF AGEING

Resource Requirements: the Government's Position

The resource demands for health and care fluctuate over the life-cycle. The average annual per capita cost of providing hospital and community health services, family practitioner services and personal social services in England in 1984–85 was £325 (HM Treasury, 1987: chart 3.14.3, p. 219). The two peak periods of resource demand over the life-cycle are birth, where the average annual cost was £1180, and towards the end of life, aged 75 years and over, where the average annual cost of NHS care was £1420. During the other parts of the life-cycle, NHS cost demands are modest: for instance, for the age group 16–64 years the average cost of care was £180.

It is these fluctuations in the cost of NHS care over the life-cycle which create public and government anxiety about the resource consequences of the ageing of the UK population. However, using these costs and the estimated increases in the number of the elderly, particularly those over 75 years of age, gives modest estimates of the expenditure increases required to fund care of the elderly in the hospital and community health services (HCHS) sector. As can be seen from Table 17.1, the effects of demography are easing and the Department of Health and Social Security may no longer be able to justify its bid to the Treasury for additional HCHS resources by using demographic arguments.

Table 17.1   Estimated growth in hospital and community health services (HCHS) budget required to meet demographic change. Source: *Hansard* (23 June 1986)

Year	Percentage increase in HCHS budget
1983–84	0.5
1984–85	0.6
1985–86	1.1
1986–87	1.0
1987–88	0.9
1988–89	0.8
1989–90	0.7
1990–91	0.6
1991–92	0.5
1992–93	0.2
1993–94	0.0
1994–95	0.1
1995–96	0.6

The Weaknesses of the Forecasting Base

However, this conclusion is dependent on the accuracy of the cost and the epidemiological data on which it is based. It is possible to constrain HCHS expenditures by aggressive policies to shorten hospital length of stay, but the effect of such actions is to shift patients on to the budgets of other carers. These carers may be publicly provided (e.g. local authority residential homes), publicly financed (e.g. private nursing homes where places are paid for out of the social security budget) or privately financed and provided. Thus, the cost data on which expenditure calculations are based are a product of the incentives faced by the fragmented system of budget holders who finance the compartmentalised system of care for the elderly. Part of this system is the informal care sector, in which spouses care for each other, neighbours provide care, and carers paid for out of, for instance, social workers' budgets combine in all sorts of ways to augment the statutory services. The costs of these inputs are often unknown, and the provision may bear little relation to client needs as measured by some dependency scale.

Not only are sectoral costs the product of the incentives operating in the caring system, they are also very difficult to estimate. Any attempt to determine the opportunity cost of particular 'packages' to care for the elderly relies on the availability of public and private sector data. The National Health Service cost data are very poor. Current costs are available only on a functional basis — i.e. the costs of medical, nursing, 'hotel' and other costs are recorded separately and on an aggregate basis. Capital costs are very difficult to compute, because until recently little effort was made to value NHS assets, let alone apportion these across different activities within a hospital.

Private sector costs — for instance, for residential and nursing home care for the elderly — are based on prices. However, prices may be greater or less than opportunity costs, and thus any costing of services based on prices may be biased upwards or downwards to an unknown degree.

Determining the costs of providing informal care is a complex task (Wright, 1987). Patients, carers and professional staff may have different perceptions of the relative costs of alternative caring modes. For instance, statutory workers may regard informal care as a 'free good', while the carers may regard the statutory services as a 'free good'. For carers (e.g. the spouse) caring is a leisure activity for some of the time, but prolonged leisure or working opportunity losses may be significant opportunity costs. The pattern of these costs will be related to the nature of the caring relationships (e.g. a spouse compared with a neighbour) and needs to be derived with care if estimates of future expenditure are to be determined with some accuracy.

Even if the cost data for statutory provision, private-sector care and informal care were robust, they have to be combined with suspect epidemiological data to provide expenditure estimates. The elderly are a very heterogeneous group, each section of which may exhibit life-cycle characteristics which differ sharply. Thus, we might expect the dependency of the rich elderly to have a different life-cycle pattern from that of the poor elderly. Also, dependence between the sexes may vary: females appear to live longer lives but the quality of the additional life-years appears to be quite poor (Silman, 1987). Indeed, like all other life-cycle events, the vicissitudes of the elderly are a product of a series of life-cycle events: initial endowments (particularly the socio-economic characteristics of parents), luck, choice and incentives. The variety of combinations of these four variables, and sub-categories within them, is immense, and thus it is inevitable that the outcomes experienced by the elderly in terms of resources and dependence is very wide.

The basic epidemiological problem is that the data about the incidence and prevalence of dependence over the life-cycle are poor. Furthermore, it is difficult to forecast future incidence and prevalence rates. Future cohorts of people arriving in old age will probably have more years of healthy lifestyles than current cohorts. This may lead to a lower incidence of chronic diseases (e.g. less smoking and less lung cancer). Furthermore, earlier diagnosis of chronic diseases and treatment together with better self-care may reverse or slow the onset of disease. Increased financial support, better rehabilitation policies and more flexible employment contracts may enable more people to cope with their disease problems and remain active with a better quality of life over a longer period of time, particularly if retirement ages are raised and people are able to remain in employment, either part- or full-time, for longer periods of time.

The consequences of such changes for future health and mortality data are complex. Mortality rates may fall and their distribution across the social classes may alter. The prevalence of killer diseases (e.g. breast cancer) could rise, owing to earlier diagnosis and reduced mortality. Declines in mortality will increase the morbidity of the population as 'survivors' live longer lives of potentially high dependence. As the benefits of earlier diagnosis begin to exhibit diminishing returns, prevalence rates may plateau or decline for killer diseases, but the rates of non-killer diseases will rise as more people survive to contract these problems. It is likely that in the short term dependence rates will continue to rise, owing to earlier diagnoses, reductions in mortality and the increased desire of individuals to care for their illnesses. In the longer term it is possible that high dependence may be less common, that partial dependence rates will rise, and that individuals may live relatively healthy lives until the multiple breakdown of the body's organs bring rapid death.

Such scenarios (developed more fully by Verbrugge, 1984) are hypotheses awaiting verification by longitudinal research. Such research is required to illuminate not only future trends, but also existing patterns of incidence and prevalence of dependence. Dependence will arise from dementia, cognitive impairment and physical disability. Cross-section research indicates that the elderly with cognitive impairment may use health care twice as much as the healthy elderly. Typically, the elderly living alone also exhibit higher levels of psychiatric distress (see, for instance, Cox *et al.*, 1987: chapter 6).

However, while there are a variety of cross-section studies in train, the extent to which they supplement knowledge is significant but incomplete. For instance, the Cambridge study (Cox *et al.*, 1987) uses a broad range of physical and behavioural measures and could contribute towards the determination of factors affecting both the risk and the rate of cognitive decline. However, this study had an overall response rate of only 60 per cent, with a response rate of less than 54 per cent for the self-completion element of the survey.

So, while cross-section studies produce results which illuminate some aspects of the life-cycle dependence characteristics of the elderly, the picture is incomplete. The only way to remedy such deficiencies is to carry out a longitudinal study, involving the regular follow-up of cohorts of the elderly over time.

The case for such a study seems strong. While the demographic structure of the elderly over the next thirty years is clear, relatively little is known about their ageing process and the factors that determine it. Improved knowledge of the factors affecting the onset of physical and cognitive decline in old age would make it possible for health and other resources to be targeted to prevent decline in health status. Without such information, the estimates of the public expenditure consequences of increasing dependence must remain largely speculative.

A longitudinal survey, particularly if it was based on multiple cohorts, could indicate survival changes for succeeding cohorts and provide the basis for better expenditure estimates and greater cost-effectiveness in the provision of services. The first 'round' of such a survey would supply 'snapshot' information for the elderly at different ages, and, if these data were linked to the General Household Survey, they could provide a wide range of data (e.g. socio-economic circumstances and use of services). Succeeding follow-ups of the same sample would indicate (at, for instance, five-year intervals) how the cognitive and physical abilities of the elderly had changed and what factors were associated with these movements.

Unless such an expensive and extensive data source is initiated, the epidemiological basis of current resource planning will continue to be incomplete at best and threadbare at worst. Fuchs (1984) estimated that the United States spends about 1 per cent of its gross national product on health care for the elderly who are in the last year of life. These costs of dying, together with the other costs associated with care of the elderly with cognitive and physical decline, mean that in all probability 40–50 per cent of health care budgets are spent on the elderly.

This cost burden, together with demographic trends, makes it sensible not only to improve the economic (costing) basis on which macro-resource consequences are measured, but also to invest in the expansion of the epidemiological stock of knowledge about the nature of cognitive and physical decline over the life-cycle and the factors which influence life-cycle trends in these variables. Without better economic and epidemiological data, the macro-economic aspects of care for the elderly will be based more on 'guesstimates' than on precise measurement of significant changes in the way in which the elderly decline into dependence. Unless such data are produced, the Finance Division of the Department of Health and Social Security will find it very difficult to substantiate their bids to the Treasury for increased spending on care for the elderly. Despite the necessity for this information, there is no indication that longitudinal surveys will be initiated. Policy at the macro level seems set to continue to be based on poor information, 'guesstimates' and assertions.

Efficient Resource Use and Care of the Elderly: Evaluation

The resource demands created by care of the elderly are substantial. Inevitably, resources are limited and care has to be rationed: acute rescue services are a clear example of this, and are discussed by Jennett in Chapter 12 of this book. If it is assumed that the objective of policy is to use resources in a cost-effective manner, it is necessary to identify the alternative forms of care available for the different elderly care groups, to cost them, to investigate their effectiveness, and then to channel resources to the most cost-effective alternatives.

A simple classification of alternative methods of caring for the elderly, together with the costs of these options, is set out in Maynard and Smith (1983). This was updated in illustrative form by the Audit Commission (1986) and is set out in Table 17.2. It can be seen that the cost of care for a frail elderly person in his or her own home was less than £100, while care in a NHS geriatric ward was nearly £300 per week.

However, although this is a simple classification mechanism which highlights the differences in the costs of alternative modes of caring for the elderly, each option covers a wide variety of different forms of provision. The levels of provision and the quality of care provided in the alternative forms of institutional and domiciliary care vary considerably, with no agreed input or activity 'norms'. Thus, any appraisal of the cost-effectiveness of the alternative has to identify carefully the characteristics of the options even before their costs or effectiveness are evaluated.

In costing the alternatives, it is essential first to identify all the opportunity costs — public and private — associated with moving the elderly from one care option to another. The costing exercise will involve seeking to place values on capital costs and current costs. These are listed in Table 17.3. Ideally, any quantification of these costs would distinguish between marginal and average costs. Most studies have produced average-cost data only and most of their authors recognise the limitations of their results.

Many studies have produced results which show domiciliary care to be cheap. Such results may have at least two defects. First, low-cost options may be poor-quality (low-provision) options. Many studies do not standardise their results by quality, and such standardisation is not easy to do — e.g. how do you measure the quality of care other than by input/process data, and is there a consensus among providers about the optimal input/process mixes? A second potential bias that may exist in cost estimates of community care is that they may omit the costs of informal care.

Table 17.2 Illustrative weekly cost (£) of alternative packages of care for an elderly person[a]. Source: Audit Commission (1986, p. 48)

	Own home	Own home + day care	LA sheltered housing	LA Part III home	P&V[b] residential home	P&V[b] nursing home	NHS geriatric ward
Cost to Social Security							
State pension	38.70	38.70	38.70	38.70	38.70	38.70	7.75
Certificated housing benefit	19.00	19.00	30.00	—	—	—	—
Attendance allowance	20.65	20.65	20.65	—	20.65	20.65	—
Supplementary benefit	1.40	1.40	1.40	—	74.70	119.70	—
Cost to NHS							
Home care	4.00	4.00	4.00	—	—	—	—
In-patient care	—	—	—	—	—	—	287.00
Cost to Personal Social Services							
Domiciliary services	12.00	12.00	12.00	—	—	—	—
Day centre	—	38.00	38.00	—	—	—	—
Residential care (net)	—	—	—	90.05	—	—	—
Cost to Housing Department							
Housing revenue account deficit on sheltered housing	—	—	5.20	—	—	—	—
Cost to DOE							
Rate relief	1.60	1.60	1.60	4.50	4.50	4.50	—
Cost by Agency							
Social Security	79.75	79.75	90.75	38.70	134.05	179.05	7.75
NHS	4.00	4.00	4.00	—	—	—	187.00
Personal Social Services	12.00	50.00	50.00	90.05	—	—	—
Housing Department	—	—	5.20	—	—	—	—
DOE	1.60	1.60	1.60	4.50	4.50	4.50	—
Total public cost	97.35	135.35	151.55	133.25	138.55	183.55	294.75

[a] Frail elderly single person on State pension (without substantial savings). Qualifying for Attendance Allowance at lower rate. Disability incurred after retirement age. Long-term costs per week.
[b] Private and voluntary.

Table 17.3 Costs to be included in the appraisal of care for the elderly. Source: Wright *et al.* (1982)

Hospital and residential care	*Community care*
Capital costs	Capital costs (housing)
Care service costs	Care service costs
General service costs	Personal living expenses
Personal consumption	Informal help

Reference has been made above to the quantification problems involved in such costs. However, if these crucial issues are omitted, substantial biases in cost estimates may be produced to confuse policy-making.

The objectives of caring policies for the elderly are listed by Challis (1981):

(1) maintenance of independence;
(2) maintenance or improvement of psychological well-being;
(3) social integration;
(4) maintenance or improvement of family relationships;
(5) development of community support;
(6) nurture (basic needs for comfort and security);
(7) compensation for disability.

Any survey (e.g. Wright, 1987) of the cost-effectiveness literature in this field generates some general conclusions. In most cases the cheapest form of care for the elderly is in their own homes, rather than in residential or nursing homes. With most people preferring to 'stay put' in their own homes, this form of care is probably cost-effective for a large majority of the elderly. The limits to such care are the self-care ability of the elderly and the availability of the support of family and friends to compensate for the increasing dependence of the elderly.

Perhaps more surprisingly, another finding from research is that there are many people with similar characteristics in all forms of care. Thus, dependence (demand) and intensity of care (supply) are poorly matched and, as if by accident, people are allocated across the compartmentalised caring system. Consequently, the residential care sector has people in it who are quite capable of caring for themselves and mobile enough to live in the community. Yet within this same sector there are people with dependence levels as high as those of patients in beds in NHS geriatric wards.

Any costing of community or institutional care is of the services offered rather than the ideal pattern of services that could be supplied. Hence, the costs may be low, and further depressed if informal care costs are ignored, and the intensity of care may be inadequate for highly dependent patients. Without active management of care intensity by, for instance, social workers, valuable opportunities for maintaining the elderly in the community may be missed. There is a growing body of evidence that high-intensity community care is cost-effective (e.g. Challis and Davies, 1986) in relation to hospital care, but its relative advantages over nursing home care are less obvious. Furthermore, the comparison of hospital care with community care does not differentiate for differing standards of hospital care.

So the comparison of provision types, in terms of costs and effects, is limited. Quality criteria are applied unevenly — e.g. District Health Authorities (DHAs) apply quality standards to private-sector nursing homes, whose owners seek the necessary NHS registration, which are superior to the standards of care provided in DHA hospitals. Domiciliary care is frequently not tailored to the dependence needs of the elderly, often because of poor case management. The elderly are not thoroughly and regularly assessed to ensure that resources are matched to needs, and there is no system to ensure that the appropriate mix of provision is provided in any locality. The problems of incomplete assessment of the costs and effects of alternative combinations of public and private, community and institutional, cash and kind, caring provision, in conjunction with the failure to appraise systematically over time the needs of patients, ensure that resources are not used efficiently.

EFFICIENT RESOURCE USE AND CARE OF THE ELDERLY: INCENTIVES

However, even if costs, needs and effectiveness were measured and monitored effectively, the problems of incentives would remain. As mentioned above, the dependent elderly are distributed in an almost random manner across the caring sector, almost regardless of needs, costs and the intensity of care. Because of the incentive system confronting the resource managers of the different components of the care system, patients are 'blocked' or discharged with little regard to cost-effectiveness criteria.

Thus, the cash-limited NHS hospital system has in-built incentives for managers to discharge patients. However, discharge policies are constrained by the provision of care in the community. For instance, the hospital manager could 'privatise' his geriatric care system by entering into arrangements with private nursing homes by which patients enter these homes, perhaps still cared for by domiciliary visits by NHS consultants, and the cost of care is met out of the social security budget.

Since the easing of the Supplementary Benefits (board and lodgings) regulations in 1981, the private nursing and residential homes sectors have grown rapidly. Only a minority (perhaps 20 per cent) of the patients in these homes are relatively independent, and even for these it is difficult to move them into possibly cheaper community care because of the lack of availability of carers in the community.

Once into institutional care, the patients may increase in dependence and the level of service provision may or may not alter to meet changing needs. Similarly, patients in the local authority institutional care sector may or may not receive care appropriate to their changing dependence over time.

At no place in the provision system is there a manager with incentives to optimise the system rather than one small part of it. No manager or policy-maker takes the system or society view: the former is concerned generally to stay within his or her cash-limited budget and the latter is concerned with his or her total or sectoral department interests.

It is not self-evident how the sectors concerned with the finance and provision of care for the elderly can be integrated in a fashion which is conducive to matching need (dependence) and provision (quality of care) at least cost. The Kent community care experiments (e.g. Challis, 1986, and Chapter 13 of this book) have allocated this role and a budget to social workers, and the early evaluative results appear encouraging in terms of both costs and effects. However, alternative professional groups — for instance, community nurses and general practitioners — are competing for the consumer-advocate budget-holder role and it is not self-evident as to which of these groups, or hospital consultant geriatricians, might carry out the task most effectively.

The diversity in practice noted by the Audit Commission (1986) forms a natural basis for experimentation and the evaluation of the costs and effects of competing methods of improving the system of care for the elderly. It is to be hoped that NHS policy-makers will fund such evaluation, so that future policy formation can be based on facts rather than 'guesstimates', prejudices and myths.

CONCLUSIONS

> 'Inspector Farnall was present and informed the Guardians that he did not think the workhouse a fit place for this class (the temporarily disabled, the aged and the infirm). He implied they should be given domiciliary relief and insinuated that the Relieving officer and the District Medical officer got rid of cases this way, because the outdoor sick cost an average of 6s, whilst workhouse in-mates only cost 3s 6d. He also said that there were only forty pauper nurses and no paid ones, these were not enough to attend the sick and the aged.'
>
> Hodkinson (1967: p. 546)

The Relieving Officer and District Medical Officer in Greenwich in 1866 responded to incentives just as managers do today. As indicated, Inspector Farnall believed that the cheapness of the workhouse option was an effect produced by a poor quality of provision, and then, as now, there was a dispute about the costs and effects of alternative care options. While we no longer separate out the sexes on entry into care as the Guardians did, decision-making continues to be fragmented, only marginally 'confused' by facts, and inefficient.

The advocacy in preceding chapters, by Karen Luker for better nursing services for the elderly, by Peter Millard for better hospital care for the elderly, by Charles Freer and Idris Williams for better primary care for the elderly, by David Hobman for increased voluntary care for the elderly, and by Muir Gray, Sheila Peace and William Laing for better living environments for the elderly, would use scarce resources and may generate substantial benefits for patients.

However, as Rex Taylor emphasises, the elderly is a heterogeneous group, and, as Bryan Jennett demonstrates unequivocally, resources are limited. It is inevitable that resources will be rationed and that some needs of the less dependent elderly will not be met. Some people will be left with physical and cognitive disabilities whose effects could be reduced by care which cannot be financed.

The objective of policy analysis must be to identify the costs and effects of competing options, so that policy-makers can identify the cost-effective mode of care for different dependence groups and induce producers and consumers to develop and use those levels of service. This requires a major break with traditions with which Inspector Farnall was familiar. The evaluation needs identified by him in 1866 continue to be unmet and result in inefficiency over 120 years later, despite continued 'redisorganisations' of the health service. Until the belief that changes in structure *per se* will resolve the inefficiencies inherent in existing practices is replaced by scientific evaluation of policy options and tested effective incentive systems, the familiar conclusions of Caius Petronius will remain apposite:

> We trained very hard, but it seemed that every time we were beginning to form up into teams, we would be reorganised. I was to learn later in life that we tend to meet any new situation by reorganising and a wonderful method it can be for creating the illusion of progress, while producing confusion, inefficiency and demoralisation.

Caius Petronius
(administrator of Emperor Nero, AD 66)

REFERENCES

Audit Commission (1986). *Making a Reality of Community Care*. HMSO, London

Challis, D. J. (1981). The measurement of outcome in social care of the elderly. *J. Social Policy*, **10** (2), 179

Challis, D. J. and Davies, L. (1986). *Case Management in Community Care*. Gower, London

Cox, B. D., Blaxter, M., Buckle, A. L. J., Golding, J. E., Gore, M., Huppert, F.A., Nickson, J., Roth, M., Start, J., Wadsworth, M. E. J. and Whichelow, M. (1987). *The Health and Lifestyle Survey: A Preliminary Report*. Health Promotion Research Trust, Cambridge

Fuchs, V. (1984). Reflections on ageing, health and medical care. *Milbank Mem. Fund Q.*, **62** (2), 143

Hodgkinson, R. G. (1967). *The Origins of the National Health Service*. Wellcome Historical Medical Library, London

Maynard, A. and Smith, J. C. (1983). *The Elderly: Who Cares? Who Pays?* Nuffield-York Portfolio 1, Nuffield Provincial Hospitals Trust, London

Silman, A. J. (1987). Why do women live longer and is it worth it? *Br. Med. J.*, **294**, 1331

HM Treasury (1987). *The Government's Expenditure Plans 1987–88 to 1989–90*, Cmnd. 56-II, Vol. 2. HMSO, London

Verbrugge, L. (1984). Longer life but worsening health? Trends in health in middle aged and older persons. *Milbank Mem. Fund Q.*, **62** (3), 475

Wright, K. G. (1987). *The Economics of Informal Care of the Elderly*. Discussion Paper 23, Centre for Health Economics, University of York

Wright, K. G., Cairns, J. and Snell, M. (1982). *Costing Care: The Costs of Alternative Patterns of Care for the Elderly*. University of Sheffield, Social Services Monograph

Conclusion

Charles Freer and Nicholas Wells

This book represents an attempt to counteract the negative attitudes that characterise much of the discussion about the elderly and the implications of future sociodemographic trends. These issues are too frequently debated in the language of crisis and impending doom. The book is based on the belief that the available evidence gives grounds for optimism about the 'greying' of the population. At the very least, it argues for a more balanced interpretation of the current and likely future situation. A wide range of contemporary issues has been examined from a number of different perspectives, and two broad themes have emerged. First, a larger proportion of the elderly population is healthier and happier than many people imagine. Second, substantial progress has undoubtedly been achieved in many of the services provided for the elderly, although much, of course, still remains to be done.

The growing awareness of the health of the elderly reflects to a large extent the contribution that gerontology has made to changing society's perspective on this age group. The focus has shifted from the abnormal and disease to the normal and the ageing process. This not only has allowed growing old to be seen in a positive light, but also has promoted a better understanding of the unique features of illness in this age group when disease and ageing interact. A further profound influence on developments in recent years has been the emergence of a life-cycle view of ageing. Retirement is not necessarily the beginning of a downhill path, but the start of a new phase of life: one with both positive and negative features, like any other stage of life, such as adolescence and middle age. Indeed, as many general practitioners will verify, it sometimes seems that other age groups — such as the 40s, with the pressures of mortgages and children growing up — have far greater life problems than the retired. As the number of old people increases, there may be attempts to formalise a subdivision between the young old and the old old. The morbidity and disability profiles of older people would appear to suggest a more appropriate cut-off point at about the age of 75 years. Such moves should, however, be resisted: they would simply shift the threshold for negative stereotyping upwards while continuing to obscure the fact that large numbers of very old people are fit and content with their lives.

The challenge for the future lies in making optimal use of the resources that are available, by ensuring that they are directed to individuals with the greatest needs. Accurate targeting of resources has never proved easy, in part because of the resistance to change that has, at least until recently, tended to prevail in the health and social services. With improvements in this respect now beginning to take place, the scope for further progress in caring for the elderly probably lies in better planning and management at the patch or neighbourhood level. At this point of entry, it is likely to be easier to diminish the barriers between services and to avoid duplication of resources. More grassroots control might also create the conditions that would encourage further experimentation with the delivery of care to find the best mix of services, given existing resources. To date, such experiments have probably been inhibited by the comprehensive and uniform nature of public services, which has also limited available choices. It is likely that a greater mix of public and private services for the elderly will be developed and that this will increase the range of care and accommodation facilities for this group without sacrificing free access to all those requiring care.

Concern for the deficiencies that clearly exist in current service provision must not be allowed to obscure the underlying strength of health and social services in Britain, or the improvements that have been described in the chapters of this book. Many richer countries still lack the comprehensive and specialist care for older people that has emerged since 1948. Services can and must be improved, but this is more likely to occur if, rather than being overwhelmed by a sense of failure, the successes of the existing system can be identified and used as a foundation for future development. A positive view will also serve to recognise the dedicated efforts of the many formal and informal carers of the elderly. Their morale must be sapped frequently in the face of a lay and professional press that seem overly attracted to 'bad news'.

Presenting a positive view of current ageing trends and their implications does not always evoke an equally positive response. This might, in part, reflect the tendency to see every human situation in the worst possible light, but it is also likely to be due to a concern that painting too positive a picture might direct attention away from individuals with very real medical and social needs. This book certainly does not attempt to minimise the significant difficulties experienced by many older people. The elderly as a group have problems, but this does not mean that they are a problem group. If society is to see the care of its older citizens as a challenge rather than a burden, a positive rather than a negative view must prevail. Furthermore, if this view was more widespread, then it is likely that older people — the fit and the frail — would feel better about themselves.

It is probably to the elderly themselves that we should return for inspiration and direction. Earlier in the book, discussion was given to the marked discrepancies between younger people's perceptions of the health and well-being of older people and the ratings of older people themselves. What explains this conflict of view? To some extent, it may reflect denial on the part of the elderly, although it also seems that self-ratings may be good predictors of morbidity and mortality as far as older people are concerned. A more likely explanation is that the outward appearances of ageing are interpreted as a reflection of health status. But health and contentment have probably a much closer correlation with self-awareness, identity and fulfilment than appearance in the mirror. Fifty-year-old individuals usually feel that they are much the same *person* as they were when they were thirty, and so with 75-year-olds. When older relatives and friends tell us that they will not go to the senior citizens' club because it is full of old people, they are not being difficult or amusing. They are saying something very important about how they see, or do not see, themselves. It is likely, however, that these self-perceptions are inhibited from full expression because older people feel that they conflict with the prevailing views of old age held by the rest of society.

Throughout history, man has had to come to terms with the phenomenon of ageing and a finite lifespan, and different cultures have varied and continue to do so in the way older people and other members of the population relate to each other. Currently in Britain, the elderly are cast in a predominantly passive and recipient role. To some extent, the success and comprehensiveness of post-war health and welfare legislation may unwittingly have contributed to this. It is probably easier and cheaper to provide services such as meals-on-wheels and home helps to the frail elderly than to encourage them to become more involved in their care. But this situation could be changing. The growing number of fit, economically secure and articulate older people may lead to a more vocal, actively involved and politicised elderly population, a development that has already occurred in the United States. The consumer input may yet be a critical factor in how attitudes to, and services for, the elderly develop.

The starting point for this book was a passage from a modern play which reflected some of society's negative views about older people. To finish on a positive note, the last word will be left to an elderly Japanese artist and writer*:

> I have been in love with painting ever since I became conscious of it at the age of six. At fifty I had published innumerable drawings but nothing I did before the age of seventy was of any value at all. At seventy-five I have at last caught nearly every aspect of nature. . . . Thus at eighty I shall have developed still further, and shall, at ninety, really enter the mystery of reality.

---

* Hokusai, preface to *A Hundred Drawings of the Fuji Yama*, 1935.

Index